COPING WITH TH

JANET HORWOOD is an ex
and journalist, specializing in h   ... a member of
the Guild of Health Writers, contributing editor to *Choice*
magazine and editor of a magazine for carers. She is also
the author of six books, including *Comfort for Depression*
and *Curing Arthritis Exercise Book* (both Sheldon Press).
She is married with three children.

To John, Joe, Rachel and Jonty

I would like to thank the many people who have helped me with the preparation of this book: the women who willingly shared their experiences of the menopause with me and helped with their comments and suggestions; my GP Dr Sara Beattie for helping me through my own menopause! At Sheldon Press, Elizabeth Marsh for kindly reading an early draft of the book; Trisha Dale for her valuable (and valued) advice and in particular my publisher, Joanna Moriarty, for so much patience and understanding. I am grateful to Dr Mike Kirby of Letchworth for sparing the time to check the medical facts and to Dr Sally Hope of the British Menopause Society for all her valuable advice and for kindly agreeing to contribute the preface.

Overcoming Common Problems

Coping with the Menopause

Janet Horwood

sheldon**PRESS**

Published in Great Britain in 2001 by
Sheldon Press
Holy Trinity Church
Marylebone Road
London NW1 4DU

British Library Cataloguing-in-Publication Data

A catalogue record for this book is available from the British Library

ISBN 0–85969–834–3

Typeset by Deltatype Limited, Birkenhead, Merseyside
Printed in Great Britain by Biddles Ltd
www.biddles.co.uk

Contents

Preface

The menopause is a natural milestone in every woman's life. Hippocrates first described the menopause in a woman of 50 years of age over 2,000 years ago. What has changed dramatically in the last century is the proportion of women reaching the menopause, and living a long and healthy life after the time our periods cease. We can now, in the twenty-first century, expect to live at least 30 years after the menopause. This is almost a third of our lives. We want to remain as active and fit as possible.

There is a bewildering array of treatments for the menopause, its symptoms, and its long-term consequences. Some of these treatments require prescriptions from doctors, but there is also an enormous market in vitamin, health food and over-the-counter preparations, as well as copious well-meaning lifestyle advice. It is a time when we want to turn over a new leaf and feel stronger in body and mind. How do we choose what is right for us?

This short and clearly written book explains the basic changes that occur at the menopause. It also lays out all the options available to you and the arguments for and against each one. Women want to stay well, but we also require the evidence to allow us to make informed decisions about our health for the future.

There has also been an enormous burst of medical interest in the post-menopausal woman. We need to know how to cut our risks of osteoporosis and heart disease. We also need to know the facts about breast cancer and deep vein thrombosis and hormone replacement therapy, and to put those risks into context. We need to understand the emotional and sexual changes that occur, and when it is safe to stop contraception. We need to know the evidence of benefit for health foods or creams before spending a lot of money.

This book has all this information, as well as the lifestyle advice that every adult should be following.

Sally Hope, FRCGP DRCOG

Introduction

The menopause is a process unique to human females. Other mammals experience something similar, but the exhaustion of their store of eggs tends to occur at the same time as the end of their lifespan, rather than just over halfway through it.

It is only relatively recently that the vast majority of women have actually lived long enough to experience a menopause – the time when the final menstrual cycle takes place. Up until the early part of the last century, those who survived to that age probably heaved a sigh of relief that they were at last released from the burdens and dangers of child-bearing. On the other hand, if the symptoms of the menopause caused her to behave 'inappropriately', a woman ran the risk of being labelled 'mad' and might even have been locked away. Most hysteria was associated with womb function, and hysterectomy was a treatment for this 'hysteria'.

Post-menopause in Western society, it was expected that, having fulfilled their function, most women would spend the remainder of their lives in the background. However, in other cultures this was when women came to the foreground. An older woman might be elevated to sit with the men or cast aside her veil, and was far more likely to be treated with a marked degree of respect as a wise woman with a great deal to offer.

The change in attitude towards the menopause is fairly recent. Our mothers and grandmothers went through this stage in their lives with very little support and even less understanding. They were often told by their doctors that symptoms such as hot flushes, overwhelming fatigue or depression were 'to be expected at your time of life'. They had to learn to live with it.

Today so much has changed. The development of HRT, not only to treat many of the symptoms of the menopause but also to benefit our health in the long term, means that instead of just regarding the menopause as an end we can realistically think of it as a beginning.

As we approach the menopause and pass through it, in our forties and fifties, we certainly don't feel old. Mostly we feel strong and well. We are ready for new challenges and experiences. There are so many possibilities – we could climb a mountain, write our first novel, change careers or partners (or both), run marathons . . . Thanks to new treatments we may even choose this time of life to start or increase our family. Or we may find that being a grandmother can be a rewarding full-time job.

However, there is a snag, because despite all the advanced thinking and medical advances we can still feel uncomfortable about this time of our lives. It seems odd that we can talk freely about sex, periods, drugs, birth and death, yet many of us feel embarrassed to mention the fact that we are passing through the menopause, let alone any of the symptoms we may be experiencing.

The reason is simple. We live in a culture dominated by stereotypes. Youth and looking young are to be admired, old age is to be dreaded. It is often mocked and laughed about, an easy target for jokes or insults. HRT may relieve many uncomfortable symptoms but it has also given us one type of model for the menopause – the forever youthful-looking celebrity when there is in fact so much more to be gained than looks. So it is hardly surprising that we start to view the menopause with dread as the first step on the slippery slope to the old age most of us don't want to reach but know we cannot avoid.

That's why so many of us still feel that the signs that the end of fertility is approaching may mean we no longer have a useful role. We begin to lose confidence. We feel we have little to offer and that no one will value us.

Understanding what is happening to us both physiologically and emotionally at this time is important. The more we know about the menopause – what is it, how it might affect us, what we can do to treat the symptoms and how we can look after ourselves – the more likely we are to be able to experience these years in a positive way.

The menopause is often compared to a second adolescence because it can be a time of turmoil, when we are no longer sure who we are or where we are going. We begin to ask the question 'Is that all there is?' We have a huge advantage over teenagers – a lifetime of experience to draw on. So, for us, the menopause can be a precious opportunity. It may be turbulent and unsettling but it also hands us the key to our second adult life, where so much is possible – and achievable.

1
What is the menopause?

The menopause is the time when a woman is no longer able to have children naturally. The ovaries have ceased to produce eggs and it has been a year since the last period. Like the majority of women you will probably begin to notice the first signs when you are in your forties, although your oestrogen levels will have started to decline several years earlier.

Put accurately, the word 'menopause' refers to the day of your last period, something most women find really hard to pin-point at the time but can look back on afterwards. The months or years leading up to this time are called the peri-menopause ('peri' means 'around', so the literal translation is 'around the end of menstruation'). But you will also hear it referred to as the change, the change of life or, less often these days, the climacteric.

In order to understand what the menopause is in medical terms, you need to look back and remind yourself of what happened right at the start of your reproductive life at puberty.

It takes about three years for the changes that take place at puberty to be completed. They start around the age of 10 when the breasts start to bud and hair appears under the armpits and around the pubis. At puberty one or two eggs begin to be produced from the ovaries each month. The eggs emerge from the ovaries, travel down one of the two Fallopian tubes and eventually arrive in the uterus (womb).

If intercourse takes place at the appropriate time, the male sperm will travel up into the Fallopian tube, and this is where fertilization may take place. If this occurs, the fertilized egg will move down into the womb, where it will cling to the lining (the endometrium) and begin to grow.

If no egg is fertilized during this stage of the monthly cycle, then the egg continues its journey into the womb and leaves the body during a period, together with the lining of the womb, which has thickened in preparation for conception.

All this activity, when periods start and stop, when eggs are released from the ovaries, is controlled by the hypothalamus, a neuroendocrine part of the brain. It produces releasing hormones, small chemicals which can travel in the bloodstream and which encourage the hormone-producing organs – for example, the breast, womb, ovary – into action. The most important gland in the

1

reproductive cycle is the anterior pituitary gland which is at the base of the skull, just below the hypothalamus.

This gland produces two further hormones, which stimulate the ovaries. Follicle stimulating hormone (FSH) ensures that at least one cell in the ovary each month develops into an egg to be released about 14 days after a period has started. It also stimulates the ovary to make oestrogen. The luteinizing hormone (LH) influences the ovary to make progesterone. These two hormones, oestrogen and progesterone, are essential for reproductive life and also play a major part in causing the symptoms so many women experience when their reproductive life starts to come to an end.

The peri-menopause

When a baby girl is born she will already have around one million eggs in her ovaries, more than she will have at puberty. By puberty the number of eggs has decreased to about 250,000, and by the time the average young woman starts to think of having children the number of eggs will be around 75,000.

The fall in numbers of eggs, due to natural decay, continues and gathers speed from your mid-thirties onwards, so that once you are in your forties there are around 5,000 eggs left. By the time of the peri-menopause, fewer than a thousand eggs are left. This is when some of the symptoms of the menopause become apparent.

In the ovaries, the few remaining follicles, which act to release the eggs, have become somewhat sluggish and seem not to respond to FSH in the same way. The pituitary gland gets the message that all is not quite as it should be, and so more FSH is produced. However, the response is erratic and so the ovary makes less and less oestrogen. The pituitary also releases more LH to encourage the ovary to make more progesterone. Occasionally levels of FSH and LH may be measured. However, they are so variable in the peri-menopause that results are not reliable, and it can be very confusing for a woman (and her GP) to find that the results of a one-off test are 'normal' and for her then to experience peri-menopausal systems.

Once you are over 45, these tests become more or less irrelevant and it makes more sense to treat the symptoms. However, in younger women, under 45, other endocrine functions as well as FSH and LH levels should also be tested, as this allows the doctor to check for infertility and a true premature menopause. Because a diagnosis of this kind of premature menopause is very devastating, the tests need to be wide-ranging to ensure accuracy.

In the average menopause, it is at around this time that you will notice a change in your periods – especially if you have been used to a regular menstrual cycle. Your periods may now become irregular; some may be heavier, others lighter; they may last for a few days or for longer than before. More often they come closer together for instance, every 20 to 21 days for several years and then further apart, occurring perhaps every six weeks.

Erratic menstruation is very often the first sign that you are entering the peri-menopause. But you may also begin to experience some of the classic symptoms of the menopause – hot flushes, a dry or itchy vagina, mood swings – many of which are due to fluctuating hormone levels. As the ovaries gradually run out of eggs, so less and less oestrogen and progesterone are produced.

However, even after egg production has ceased, some oestrogen, as well some other useful hormones, continues to be produced by the ovaries and by the adrenal glands. The other hormones include the male hormones testosterone and androsteindione.

Androsteindione is converted in the adrenal glands and in fat tissue into oestrone, a weaker version of the female hormone oestrogen. The amount produced does vary, but in many women it will be enough to prevent or at least lessen some of the effects of the loss of oestrogen, such as maintaining activity in the glands in the vagina so it is less likely to atrophy, keeping the skin lubricated and reducing hair loss. However, if too much oestrogen continues to be produced – and this tends to happen in women who are overweight and have a lot of fat tissue – there is a higher risk that cancer of the womb or breast cancer can develop.

Testosterone, which is also produced by the adrenal glands, may lead to thinning hair on the scalp and pubis, an increase in facial hair and smaller breasts. However, on the plus side, testosterone can encourage enthusiasm and helps your ability to continue to enjoy sex during the years following the menopause.

Once the menopause has been reached, everything begins to settle down. As the levels of FSH and LH gradually reduce, you should experience fewer uncomfortable symptoms.

The vital hormones

Hormones are chemical substances produced principally by the endocrine glands, under the brain's direction, and released into the bloodstream. There they act as messengers, telling other organs to make different chemicals to produce a specific effect. It is thanks to hormones that an efficient control system is maintained within the body, ensuring that basic functions such as temperature regulation, blood pressure, blood sugar levels and heart rate work properly and can also adjust to changing circumstances. Hormones can affect our mood, our overall health and our ability to perform well.

The sex hormones play a vital role in our lives, enabling both men and women to develop the sexual characteristics that regulate sperm and egg production and the menstrual cycle, preparing us for reproduction. For women there are two main types of hormone – oestrogens and progestogens, or progesterone.

Oestrogen

In order to ovulate, the ovaries produce a hormone called oestrogen – this production starts a few years after puberty. The amount produced increases during the cycle to reach a peak around 12 days after a period has started. Oestrogen also encourages the womb lining to thicken, sends messages back to the pituitary gland and affects breast development. During the time when conception might take place, oestrogen also ensures that the mucus which lines the vagina and keeps it moist is stretchy and clear. The mucus acts like a net to help sperm scramble up through the cervix to the womb.

Oestrogen also has many other roles, and lack of it does have long-term effects. As oestrogen levels fall during the menopause, changes begin to take place within a woman's body. The majority of these changes are quite minor and not at all life-threatening. However, they are noticeable, and bearing in mind all the other changes that can be taking place around this time in your life, it's easy to become distressed about them. What can help is knowing why all this is happening and what it all means. In some cases you can take some action to prevent or lessen the effects.

Vagina and bladder

Low oestrogen levels are particularly noticeable in the effect they have on skin cells. Internally, the cells that line the vagina, the bladder and the urinary tract lose their elasticity and may become dry and thinner. This can make intercourse painful and you may be more likely to develop an infection such as cystitis. Many women also suffer from itching and soreness in the area. Hormone replacement therapy (HRT) can help relieve these symptoms in the vagina and urethra, but you can also relieve many uncomfortable vaginal symptoms with pessaries or creams containing oestrogen or by using a gentle water-based lubricant such as KY Jelly.

Skin

Outwardly you will begin to notice changes in your skin. Wrinkles will become more apparent, the skin around the jaw-line and neck may begin to sag, and your skin may also become very dry.

Many women spend a small fortune on lotions, potions and beauty treatments to try and halt the ageing process. Most studies have shown that creams have little effect, and beauty salon treatments have to be kept up for the slight difference to be maintained. Only cosmetic surgery can change the look of your skin for a while.

However, you can do a great deal to improve your skin by applying a moisturizer day and night. Eating well and taking regular exercise will also help to give your skin a healthier appearance (despite the lines). Staying out of the sun will not only prevent more lines, it will also protect your skin against further damage. Even on a cloudy day it is advisable to use either a sunscreen or a moisturizer with a sun protection factor (SPF) of a minimum of 12. Finally – stop smoking! There is good evidence that smokers have more and earlier wrinkles than non-smokers. Also, if you smoke, your menopause is likely to occur two years earlier.

Hair

You will notice as you go through the menopause that your hair texture changes. The hair on your head becomes finer and thinner and may be more difficult to handle, and there is also some loss of pubic hair. Meanwhile body hair appears in places you would much prefer it didn't, such as on the face, particularly on the chin and upper lip. This is due to the increase in male sex hormones such as testosterone; for some women it can become very embarrassing, as the fine hair that normally covers all our bodies can change into much darker, coarser hair and be visible on the chest and stomach as well as the face and arms.

Increasing oestrogen levels by taking HRT can reduce these problems, and there are also effective beauty treatments to remove unwanted facial hair.

Heart

It's only relatively recently that the protective role of oestrogen in reducing the risk of heart disease among women has begun to be recognized. However, there is some controversy surrounding this because of a parallel increased risk of blood clots forming and causing deep vein thrombosis. Although we have yet to understand exactly what happens after the menopause (or hysterectomy or surgical removal of the ovaries), there is no doubt that once oestrogen ceases to be produced a woman's risk of heart attack is equal to a man's and becomes the most common cause of death.

One of the signs to watch out for is an increase in cholesterol levels. Scientists have discovered that once the ovaries cease to function, there is a rise in low-density cholesterol (LDL), known as the 'bad' cholesterol, but a decrease in high-density cholesterol (HDL), which is known to protect the heart.

Muscles and joints

At the same time the muscles of the body are beginning to lose strength and stamina. This is the time to start exercising to maintain good muscle tone and balance and avoid falls and weakness later in life. Collagen, which joints need as a lubricant, is also in short supply now, so it's important to keep moving to ensure your joints retain their mobility. Oestrogen acts on collagen to keep it springy – so the muscles and ligaments of the pelvic floor can begin to sag post-menopause and cause the womb/rectum/bladder to drop. To prevent a prolapse it's important to keep the pelvic floor muscles well toned.

Bones

During the menopause the balance of bone health is disturbed, although a deterioration in bone turnover will have been present for some years before the menopause. Normally the two types of cell involved – osteoblasts and osteoclasts – work in harmony. The former builds up bone while the latter removes it. During and after the menopause the osteoclasts become very active so more bone is removed than replaced, and as a result bone becomes more porous and loses its density and strength.

At the same time, lack of oestrogen makes it harder for the body to use the vitamins and minerals that are essential for good bone health. Bone-building vitamins such as vitamin D and minerals such as calcium are harder to absorb. The hormone calcitonin, which regulates the amount of calcium in the body, is used less efficiently and more calcium is lost, putting bones at risk of fracture.

Breasts and stomach

The size and shape of your breasts will begin to change, and unfortunately, because there are no muscles in the breasts, exercise will not restore them to their former fullness. Breast tissue also changes due to lack of oestrogen, and as a result there is less glandular tissue and more fat.

However, you can do something about an increase in the size of your waist at this stage in your life. Keep a balance between how much you eat and how much you exercise. Metabolism slows as we age and this means that unless you are taking plenty of exercise you won't be burning off the same amount of calories. If at the age of 48 you continue to eat as much as you did at 38, you will put on weight. The answer is to eat a little less and exercise regularly. Abdominal exercises will give you a flatter stomach and also build up the muscles needed to support the back. Have good amounts of fibre in your diet and drink plenty as well, especially water.

Brain

There are oestrogen receptors in many sites in the brain – for instance in the hippocampus, which is where we store a great deal of information and which is responsible for our ability to remember things. Research is still continuing into how lower oestrogen levels may affect these receptors and, in turn, the way women function emotionally and intellectually at the menopause.

One line of research has established that oestrogen is a natural tranquillizer that can help us to feel less anxious and worried.

Although HRT can relieve these symptoms, the secret is to keep your mind well exercised and challenged. Adopt a 'use it or lose it' philosophy and continue to do crosswords, read, enjoy stimulating company and events, learn new skills and adopt different ideas and approaches.

Progesterone

Once ovulation has taken place, even if an egg has not been fertilized oestrogen production increases again and another hormone, progesterone, is produced. This also thickens the womb lining, making it even softer and more sponge-like and creating tiny hollows where a fertilized egg can find a safe place to grow.

Progesterone also has an effect on vaginal mucus, which now becomes thicker so that further sperm are discouraged from getting into the Fallopian tubes. Both hormones work together, causing the tubes to expand and contract and enable the egg to move smoothly on its way to the uterus, which takes between six and seven days.

If the egg has not been fertilized, on about the twenty-eighth day of the monthly cycle production of these two hormones falls quite sharply and this triggers the shedding of the womb lining – in other words, the normal bleeding of a period. When hormone levels fall there may be other symptoms such as breast tenderness, mood swings, fluid retention – the classic symptoms of pre-menstrual syndrome (PMS). As you look back from the menopause you will realize that suffering regularly from PMS was in many ways like having a miniature menopause each month.

How will I know if this is the real thing?

It is impossible to know beforehand exactly when your menopause will occur, but the average age for the menopause in Britain is between 48 and 55. There has been some research to show that the age you begin to menstruate may be linked to the age you experience the menopause, and many women experience the menopause at the same age as their mothers did. If you had an early puberty you may have an earlier menopause than someone who began menstruating later but this is by no means proven.

Most women will know when they are entering the menopause from symptoms and the way they feel. As previously mentioned, blood tests to show levels of oestrogen and progesterone are not particularly reliable or even necessary.

In most cases you won't need blood tests to show hormone or FSH levels. But 1 per cent of 40-year-old women do experience premature ovarian failure. If you are under 45 and experiencing a number of unexplained symptoms and would normally not expect to be menopausal at your age, you should ask to be referred to a specialist clinic.

An early menopause

If menopausal symptoms begin to occur before you are 45, it is now accepted that you are experiencing a premature or early menopause. There are several reasons for this.

- Some women are simply born with fewer eggs in their ovaries.
- If you have had chemotherapy for any cancer or radiation treatment for pelvic cancer, there is a chance that many eggs will have been destroyed.
- Viral illnesses such as mumps can damage eggs.
- It is possible that stress, heavy smoking (smokers experience the menopause on average two years earlier) or drinking and heredity can also play a part in reducing the number of eggs.
- Auto-immune diseases such as rheumatoid arthritis can sometimes

cause the body to produce antibodies which attack the ovaries and destroy the eggs in them.

- Surgery. A hysterectomy can be performed in several ways depending on the reasons for the operation.

A partial hysterectomy means that the uterus (womb) and cervix (neck of the womb) are removed but the ovaries and Fallopian tubes are left intact. Oestrogen continues to be produced and ovulation takes place, but there is no period. Younger women who have had this operation have a higher (30 per cent) chance of experiencing an early menopause.

A total hysterectomy will involve removal of the ovaries and Fallopian tubes as well. This automatically triggers an early menopause. The sudden drop in oestrogen levels, compared to the slow decline experienced during the average menopause, can produce very severe symptoms – both physical and emotional. Hormone replacement therapy (HRT) is prescribed to deal with these symptoms.

When the early menopause is not induced by surgery, the symptoms are sometimes different from those of the average menopause, so it is often some time before a correct diagnosis is made. Although you may experience hot flushes and other classic symptoms, you may not attribute them to the menopause. The main clue that things are changing is irregular periods, and this is the reason why most younger women finally see their doctor.

At this stage a doctor is far more likely to assume other reasons for unpredictable periods – pregnancy, dramatic weight loss (perhaps due to crash dieting), being excessively overweight, taking too much exercise or even something quite simple such as stress. These possibilities have to be eliminated before the suggestion that the woman might be experiencing premature menopause can be tested.

The main test used at this stage will be a blood test to measure hormone levels, not just FSH but LH and prolactin. At the same time the doctor will probably also take samples to assess thyroid function, as a thyroid disorder can often affect your periods. If the results suggest that you are indeed menopausal, then you may be referred to a gynaecologist for further tests to establish exactly why this is occurring – whether it is simply due to a lack of eggs or has some other cause. An ultrasound examination will give a clear view of the ovaries and of whether there are any cysts or other diseases.

Once the diagnosis has been confirmed, hormone replacement treatment is often suggested, because lack of the hormone oestrogen puts a younger woman at higher risk of developing osteoporosis or heart disease as she will have lost the protective effects of oestrogen so much earlier.

It can be tremendously difficult for a young woman to come to terms with an early menopause and the knowledge that she can no longer have children at an age when she would normally continue to be fertile.

These days a younger woman who hopes to start a family or have more children does have some options. Drugs used for fertility treatment, such as clomiphene, are now available to stimulate ovulation. If this is not successful then egg donation may be another possibility if you still have a womb; once fertilization with your partner's sperm has taken place in a test-tube, one or two embryos may be placed in the womb, while others may be frozen for use later in case this first treatment is unsuccessful.

Whatever decision is made, the most important treatment of all for early menopause is counselling.

It was really like a bereavement, except I wasn't mourning the loss of a child but the loss of all the children I would now never be able to have. We considered IVF but it's expensive and we knew that the failure rate was high. It put a tremendous strain on our marriage, and in the end I went for counselling, and later Bob joined me at the sessions because, of course, he also had lost something precious.

A late menopause

It is mainly women who are overweight who may find they are having a late menopause. If you are over 55 and are still having periods this can be perfectly normal, but it is still worth having a check-up to make sure that all is well. There is a down side to a late menopause – the fact that your body is producing oestrogen for longer may increase your risks of developing breast or uterine cancer. Here again, making sure you check your breasts regularly, going for a mammogram every three years and having a regular smear test and pelvic examination are sensible precautions.

Contraception

Throughout the peri-menopause, it is important to remember that you are still fertile and can therefore get pregnant. This suits some women, but not every woman wants to start or add to her family in her mid to late forties or even in her early to mid fifties. If you have always used the oral contraceptive pill, the synthetic oestrogen in it will help reduce the symptoms caused by the falling levels of natural oestrogen. Or you may prefer to use a progestogen-only pill, which is taken every day, to prevent ovulation. If you choose to take HRT, remember that this is not a contraceptive as the amounts of oestrogen are much lower. So you need to use reliable contraception as well.

If you are married or in a stable relationship you may decide to switch to a different form of contraception such as the diaphragm or condoms. Some women may choose to have an intra-uterine contraceptive device (IUCD). This works well for many mature women, although if your periods become very heavy it may have to be removed. However, new types of IUCD such as levornorgestrel (Mirena coil) provide contraceptive protection for three years before needing to be replaced. There is the advantage of no periods, and it can also be used as the progestogenic part of HRT.

Since you will still be going for regular check-ups of your method of contraception, you will be able to discuss what you might use during the peri-menopause with a family planning counsellor, the practice nurse or your own GP. Experts agree that if you are aged between 45 and 50 you should continue to use some form of contraception for two years after your last period. If you are over 50, this can be reduced to one year.

Is it the menopause?

Physical symptoms	none	mild	moderate	severe
Hot flushes				
Night sweats				
Palpitations (fast heartbeats)				
Irregular periods				
Stress incontinence				
Vaginal dryness				
Vaginal irritation				
Weight gain				
Hair and skin thinner				
Headaches				
Loss of muscle tone				
Fatigue/joint pains				
Constipation/IBS				
Periodontal (gum) disease				
Psychological symptoms				
Insomnia				
Poor memory/ concentration				
Depression				
Anxiety				
Decreased libido (sex drive)				
Mood swings				

Score:

0 for no symptoms
1 for mild symptoms
2 moderate symptoms
3 for severe symptoms

0–6: Pre-menopausal score – these mild symptoms could be due to other factors. See your doctor to discuss these symptoms, especially if they are affecting your lifestyle or if they are persistent or get worse. Simply making adjustments to your diet and lifestyle may help, or the doctor may be able to suggest other treatments.

7–13: Enough symptoms for the menopause to be affecting your quality of life. Go for well-woman screening, talk to your doctor.

14–20: These symptoms are more severe and are probably really affecting your ability to cope on a daily basis. Again, see your doctor to discuss possible treatments.

21 and above: Only a minority of women experience the sort of menopause that really turns their lives upside down, and you are among them. HRT can be very helpful if you are experiencing such a wide range of severe symptoms, but here again, you may prefer to adopt the natural approach.

2

What's happening to your body?

Some women do sail through their menopause without even noticing. But for every woman who has no symptoms at all, there are others who suffer really badly from menopausal symptoms that last for years and turn their lives upside down. However, most women will have some symptoms that make their lives uncomfortable, and at times it may feel as if you no longer know yourself or your body.

The majority of the physical symptoms of the menopause – the hot flushes, night sweats, irregular periods – are the result of the hormonal changes that are taking place. Oestrogen levels do not tail off slowly and evenly: they can fluctuate quite dramatically before finally settling to their lower level, as can levels of other hormones linked to the reproductive system – progesterone, FSH and LH.

There are also other changes that take place within the body around this time that are believed to be the result of lowered or erratic levels of hormones. These can include bladder problems such as leakage of urine and infections, and aching muscles and joints. Even responsibility for weight gain, thinning hair and ageing skin can be laid at the door of declining hormone levels.

The main symptoms

Hot flushes

These are the most common symptoms of all, experienced by over 80 per cent of women to a greater or lesser extent. For many, hot flushes will occur during the two years around the time of their final period, and for some they will continue for up to five years after the menopause. For a small minority, hot flushes can continue for ten years or more after the menopause.

The sensation is quite unique, and nothing like the sort of sweat you work up during exercise or when lying in the sun. For many the worst aspect of these flushes is their unpredictability – there is no time to prepare for a hot flush, for mostly they just come out of the blue. At other times they may come during exercise or if you make an extra physical effort – for instance, washing the floor. Some women also experience hot flushes when they get upset or tense.

I would be sitting there in a meeting and suddenly I'd feel it start. There would be no time to do anything – it literally happened within seconds of that first sensation of warmth and a feeling of pressure spreading around my head, neck and upper body. I know that I didn't go red, although it felt as if I did, but sweat would trickle down my face and between my breasts. They never lasted for long, but on bad days I'd have a hot flush every hour.

This sudden rise in body temperature affects the whole body from the tips of the toes to the top of the head, although it is normally felt mainly around the face and neck. Some women will flush and go red in the face and neck, others will simply perspire and feel sweat trickling down their backs, under their arms, between their breasts. Most women can feel their heart beating faster, and some can suffer from palpitations or headaches. In really bad cases, hot flushes can occur as often as five or six times an hour, throughout the day. Most flushes last for around three minutes, and it's quite normal to go from feeling completely overheated to feeling quite cold and shivery.

The reasons
The precise causes of hot flushes are not yet known, but it is believed that they occur as the result of mixed messages being received by the brain about the body's temperature.

The hypothalamus controls the body's temperature. When it believes the body temperature to be too high, it sends messages to dilate (widen) the blood vessels to increase the amount of blood flowing beneath the surface of the skin. For some reason, during the menopause the hypothalamus is less reliable. During a hot flush this increase in blood flow is quite dramatic and is accompanied by an increase in pulse and heart rate.

What you can do
Hot flushes do seem to occur more often in summer or in warm conditions, so the advice for clothing (below) is even more useful during the warmer months of the year.

Hormone replacement therapy can help control hot flushes quite successfully. In some cases relief is experienced after a couple of weeks, but mostly it will take around three months before the full benefits are felt. Dixarit, a tablet which is used to treat high blood pressure, can be helpful in reducing hot flushes. It works by making the blood vessels less likely to relax and dilate.

There are several things you can do for yourself which will at least reduce the discomfort of the hot flushes when they occur.

- It helps to dress in layers, making it easier to take things off during a flush and put them back on again afterwards. Choose clothes made from natural fabrics such as cotton or linen rather than synthetics such as polyester, as these will cling to you when you perspire. It can also help to keep the neck clear, so avoid roll-neck jumpers, clothes that button up to the chin or scarves round the neck. Choose loose-fitting blouses, scooped or V-neck jumpers.
- If you are in a public place when the flush occurs, simply take off a layer of clothing until it has passed. If you have to attend a lot of meetings you might consider taking a battery-operated fan with you (although some women would feel this simply draws attention to what is going on!) and drink plenty of cold water. If you are at home, it's much easier to fling off your clothes and even have a cool shower.
- Relax about the flushes if you possibly can – some women say they experience more hot flushes when they are stressed. When you feel one coming, try to breathe slowly and deeply throughout, and you may find it reduces the intensity of the flush.
- Watch what you eat. Certain foods seem to trigger hot flushes, so avoid spicy foods, alcohol and drinks that contain caffeine, such as tea, coffee and colas. Cut down on sugar and salt and drink plenty of plain water.
- Stop smoking – nicotine does affect the circulation and is believed to increase the likelihood of hot flushes.
- Take plenty of exercise. Some studies have shown that women who exercise regularly have fewer hot flushes.

Night sweats

Again, not every woman will experience night sweats – having hot flushes during the day does not mean you will have sweats at night, although women who have night sweats do tend to have hot flushes as well.

Night sweats are similar to hot flushes but they are often much stronger.

I would wake in the night absolutely drenched with sweat, and once or twice a week I would have to change the sheets, especially during the summer when it was warmer. The trouble was that the night sweats completely ruined my sleeping pattern, so that even when I didn't have the sweats I was still waking up several times a night.

What you can do
As with hot flushes, the key is to try and keep your surroundings as cool as possible.

- Make sure your bed linen and night clothes are made of cotton rather than nylon, polyester, silk or satin, as these fabrics tend to cling to the body. You may find it more comfortable to sleep in the nude. Sleep under several light layers of sheets and blankets rather than one or two thick layers. If you use a duvet, always have a sheet and maybe a thin blanket between yourself and the duvet. When you get warm you can fling off the duvet but run less risk of getting chilled if you still have a sheet and thin blanket to cover you.
- Have a small bowl of water, a flannel and a hand towel by your bed to cool yourself down, and a jug or bottle of fresh water to replace the fluids lost through sweating.
- Keep the bedroom well aired, even in winter. It's better to have more bed coverings than to keep the heating on in the bedroom at night. It's also a good idea to have a window open most nights to allow fresh air to circulate.
- Use relaxation exercises when you get to bed to unwind completely before going to sleep. If you wake in the night, repeat the exercises; even if you don't fall asleep again for a while, you will be resting.

Insomnia

As well as the sleep problems often caused by night sweats, you may find that during the menopause you find it harder to get to sleep, or you may start to experience broken nights – waking several times a night. Low oestrogen levels also seem to affect the quality of sleep, so that even if you don't wake up during the night, you may not feel as rested as you used to in the morning, and really have to make an effort to get out of bed and get yourself going.

Broken sleep or poor sleep has a knock-on effect. You can end up over-tired, irritable, stressed and depressed. Lack of sleep may reinforce many of the negative feelings you have about yourself as you go through the menopause, so it's important to try and sort something out if you are losing sleep. If you are married or living with someone, then your constant tossing and turning and the heat you exude will naturally also affect them.

What you can do

If your insomnia is triggered by night sweats then try some of the remedies listed above. If you are not sure why you are not sleeping, it is worth seeing your doctor and discussing possible causes with her – these could be emotional or medical, and in either case she may be able to suggest appropriate medication or treatment.

Before taking any medication such as sleeping pills or anti-depressants which your doctor may mention, try some self-help measures.

- Make preparation for bedtime as relaxing as possible. For at least an hour before you go to bed, gradually wind down from the pressures and demands of the day. Have a warm but not hot bath, keep the lighting in the bedroom low, and when you go to bed listen to some music or a favourite audio book rather than the late-night news.
- If you have had a very bad night, try not to sleep during the day. It's a good idea to keep to a routine and always go to bed at more or less the same time.
- Some women find a warm drink helpful. Milk is good last thing at night but you should avoid anything with caffeine, so no hot chocolate!
- Don't exercise in the evening. Although some experts claim it can make you feel tired, in fact it can also liven you up. If you are exercising regularly then do so in the morning, afternoon or early part of the evening. In the evening the best form of 'exercise' is relaxation, some gentle stretches or making love with your partner.
- Take a long, hard look at your mattress. If it's more than ten years old, it's time to get a new one. If you have back problems then you will need to choose carefully. Most people know they should avoid soft mattresses, but an extra hard mattress can be equally uncomfortable as it offers no support for the spine. If you share a bed with someone, you could consider buying a split mattress so that you disturb each other less in the night and also have plenty of extra space.
- When you wake in the night, try not to worry about the fact that you are losing sleep. If you don't feel too wide awake, simply lie quietly in the bed, on your back or side, and rest. If you feel you

can't drift off to sleep again it makes sense to get up for a while read a book, do some sewing or knitting before returning to bed.
- Try some of the natural remedies mentioned in Chapter 7.

Vaginal dryness

Lower oestrogen levels make the vagina drier, and the lining becomes much thinner. This lack of lubrication can make sexual intercourse painful, and this in turn leads to the myth that women no longer enjoy sex after the menopause. Physiologically your libido may also be affected by the drop in hormones.

The truth is that if intercourse is uncomfortable then you are psychologically less likely to want to make love – and of course there may well be other factors in your life and relationship with your partner that affect your libido.

However, on a purely physiological level, if the lack of lubrication can be dealt with, many women find they enjoy sex just as much, if not more, than before – with the fear of pregnancy ruled out.

It is important to keep the area lubricated, as a dry vagina makes the whole genital area much more prone to itching, soreness and infections.

What you can do

- If you see your doctor she may well suggest HRT as a way of dealing with vaginal dryness, but there are also oestrogen creams that can be applied locally. If you prefer you can buy vaginal gels over the counter at the chemist and use these to moisturize the area. The gel is designed to cling to the walls of the vagina, so one application will last up to four days and the gel can be used twice a week.
- Regular intercourse or masturbation will help to keep the vagina healthy and encourage natural lubrication.
- Use a water-based jelly such as KY Jelly before you make love, and don't use any creams, powders or perfumes on the vagina, as they may irritate it. This also includes being careful what you put in the bath in the way of scented foams and bubbles, and not washing the genital area with soap or some shower gels.

Aches and pains

It is often as a woman approaches the menopause that she begins to experience symptoms such as pains in her joints or her back, or discomfort in her stomach and bowels. These are common signs of the menopause and are in part due to lowered oestrogen levels. What they are not, in most cases, is what you must expect to put up with as you age!

Lack of oestrogen triggers a reduction in collagen. These protein fibres support muscles, joints and the connective tissues. With less collagen you are more likely to experience pain in your joints and muscles. This is not the result of over-use of joints which leads to osteoarthritis, so you need not be afraid to continue to exercise. In fact, it's even more important now to continue to work to strengthen muscles and keep joints supple.

However, frequent pains in the joints or muscles should always be checked, so see your doctor. A common problem for women in mid-life is carpal tunnel syndrome. This may start with numbness or pins and needles in the fingers and hands and up the arms. It is due to water retention and the narrowing of the passageway in the wrist which contains nerves taking messages from the brain to the hand. Carpal tunnel syndrome can be very painful if there is pressure on the nerves, and the doctor may prescribe a diuretic to get rid of excess water and an anti-inflammatory drug. Rest is helpful, and you may have to wear splints on the wrists at night for a while. Sometimes a simple steroid injection into the carpal tunnel relieves symptoms. In rare cases surgery may have to be performed to open the tunnel and free the nerve.

The digestive system

Constipation is quite common at this time, even if you have always been regular and eat sensibly. Oestrogen does play a role in keeping bowel movements regular, so with less of it around you may find that your motions will become less frequent and your stools will be harder, drier and smaller.

The other problem many women complain about is bloating and wind.

> It was really bizarre. In the morning, when I woke up, my stomach would be quite flat and comfortable, but by lunchtime it would have swollen considerably so that clothes would begin to feel tight. In the afternoon I would have a lot of wind but that didn't seem to affect the size of my stomach – I had to wait until the following morning for it to reduce in size again.

The best solution for constipation, before you resort to laxatives, is to eat a diet high in fibre, especially from fresh fruit and vegetables.

Figs and prunes are a traditional stand-by that will work for many women, but alongside the fibre it's essential to drink plenty of fluids, preferably plain mineral water. Tea and coffee are both diuretics, so even several cups of tea will have little effect in moisturizing the intestines. Two litres of water a day is recommended to keep the system working well. Rather than having a two-litre bottle at your side, try drinking this in small glasses – you will find that eight or nine will give you the amount of water you need.

For stomach bloating and wind, some experts suggest that cutting down on foods that cause fermentation in the stomach, such as yeast either in yeast extract, breads or pizzas and sugar, can help.

If you are on HRT this may also cause bloating if the oestrogen dose is too high for you. On the other hand, because progesterone is known to cause constipation and fluid retention, you may need to adjust this dose as well.

Bladder problems

The urinary tract has similar problems to the vagina in that it becomes thinner and drier during the menopause. At this time you may become more vulnerable to bladder infections such as cystitis, an inflammation of the bladder, and thrush.

Many women first experience incontinence problems during pregnancy or after childbirth, when the pelvic muscles lose their strength due to straining. This may recur at the menopause due to lack of collagen in the skin, which up until now has supported the pelvic organs such as the bladder and bowel. There may also be a prolapse of the uterus when the ligaments that support the uterus and the vagina become weaker. Your womb drops, and you get the feeling that something is coming down into the vagina.

Stress incontinence

This is the most common type of incontinence – around 40 to 50 per cent of women experience this at some stage in their lives. For some the slightest pressure will make the bladder leak, while for the majority leakage will occur when they are being active – exercising vigorously or carrying something heavy. Stress incontinence easily disrupts everyday activities such as laughing, coughing or sneezing.

I first noticed the problem at my aerobics class. At first it was just a tiny dribble, barely noticeable, but it got worse and in the end I had to stop going. I was so embarrassed.

Urge incontinence

Getting the signs that you need to pass water almost at the same time as you actually do so, is very upsetting and embarrassing. Regular visits to the toilet can help avoid accidents. Gradually increase the length of time between visits and make sure your bladder is completely empty each time.

Underactive bladder

If you store urine for too long you may develop a urinary tract infection. The bladder may become permanently distended and leakage from the overfull bladder may occur.

How to cope

Many women try to cope on their own without seeking help. They go to the toilet frequently and use sanitary towels to hide occasional leaks. They live in dread of an 'accident' and become very concerned that they may smell of urine.

It may help if you realize how many others there are like you going through the same problems and yet too embarrassed to seek help. A survey in one GP practice near Oxford showed that 30 per cent of menopausal women experienced urinary problems, but they had not mentioned it because they were too embarrassed. If you can possibly pluck up the courage to see your doctor, you will be relieved to find that you are not unusual and that you can be helped in various ways. Once the problem has been assessed, you will probably be referred to a local continence advisor.

If you really cannot bring yourself to talk to your GP, then there is an excellent Continence Advice Line (national helpline: 020 7831 9831 (all calls confidential); website: www.continence-foundation. org.uk).

Helping yourself

- Drink plenty of water – about two litres in 24 hours is needed for a healthy bladder and bowel. A glass or two of cranberry juice may help reduce the risk of urinary infections, but tea, coffee, alcohol and sugary drinks such as colas may irritate the bladder.
- Until the problem is resolved, you will need to plan outings carefully, checking toilet facilities along your route.
- Don't hesitate to see a continence advisor or local support group.
- While the incontinence is difficult to control, look at the range of continence wear available. There is no need to buy sanitary towels or cut up hand towels at home, although some people still prefer

to use terry nappies. These days there are pads of all kinds both disposable and washable and ranges of reusable underwear, cushion covers and portable urinals for men and women.

- If stress incontinence is the problem then learn to do pelvic floor exercises (see p. 24).

Your doctor may well offer you HRT, but if you have no other major menopausal symptoms you should be able to improve things considerably with physiotherapy. This will include regular pelvic floor exercises. You need to be patient, as it will take between three and six months before you notice any real change and the exercises will need to be continued long-term to sustain the improvement.

If you are finding it hard to identify the pelvic floor muscles, weighted vaginal cones can be supplied by your continence advisor. These are inserted rather like tampons, and they come in different weights. The idea is to start off with the lightest weight, insert it into the vagina and, by using your pelvic floor muscles, prevent it from falling out. Once you can hold in the lightest weight, you can progress until you can hold on to the heaviest cone. This type of 'weight lifting' can be very helpful if your main problem is poor muscle tone.

The advisor may suggest using electrical treatment, which provides stimulation to the muscles to increase the tone. Some of the equipment can be used at home once you have been taught how to use it. As well as making the muscles contract for you, it helps you to be more aware of which muscles are involved and to progress towards doing the exercises yourself. Biofeedback techniques can also help identify the correct muscles and monitor progress.

In some cases, surgical procedures may be needed to treat the problem. Some are quite simple – for instance, collagen can be injected into a weakened bladder neck – but other procedures do involve surgery and stitches. For example, if there has been a prolapse it will need to be repaired. A prolapse occurs when the ligaments that support the womb, bowel and bladder are damaged through straining. The main cause usually goes back to childbirth, but it can occur at menopause through straining due to chronic constipation or being overweight. There may also be a family history of this type of problem, and your collagen might be weak through genetic differences.

Finally, there are a number of devices on the market that can help contain any leakage while the problem is being treated. Most are disposable, and although at the moment you should discuss this with a continence advisor, it is possible that in future a number of the simpler devices that do not need to be checked and sized, such as vaginal sponges, may become available over the counter at chemists.

How to do pelvic floor exercises
These exercises were developed by Arnold Kegel to strengthen the pelvic muscles following childbirth, but they are also excellent for the vagina, making it more sensitive as well. The exercises can be performed anywhere – sitting, standing or lying down, waiting for the bus or train, in a traffic jam – and no one will ever know you are doing them. You can do them during sexual intercourse to stimulate and increase arousal. They are one of the best ways to treat incontinence.

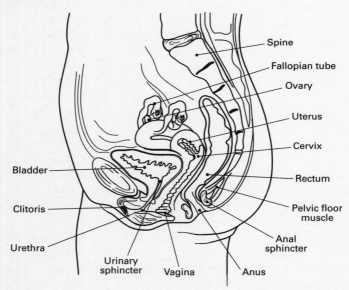

The first step is to know which muscle you are supposed to be exercising. The best way to do this is on the loo. As you pass water, try to stop the flow in mid-stream. You may find this a little hard to do at first and some urine may continue to trickle through, but the more you practise the easier it will become. You should eventually be able to stop your urine completely in mid-flow and you will know the sensation experienced by pulling up the pelvic floor muscles.

Do these exercises twice a day to start with – squeezing and releasing 10 to 15 times. Try not to squeeze the thigh or stomach muscles at the same time. At first you may find it easier to do the exercises lying on the floor or with a cushion underneath your bottom. Once this feels comfortable you can increase the exercise to five or six times a day, and then progress to holding the squeeze for three to five seconds before relaxing and repeating. After a month or so of exercising, you should begin to notice a difference.

Men can also benefit from these exercises; once learned, they can use them to control ejaculation and increase sexual pleasure.

Painful or lumpy breasts

Like the rest of your body, your breasts are also changing. They lose their fullness and may start to sag – this will be more noticeable if your breasts are large. The nipples get smaller, as well.

For most women, however, the look of their breasts is less important than the way they feel. If you have regularly suffered from sore, full and tender breasts before your period, you will recognize the sensation. This discomfort can become even more common in the peri-menopause and at the menopause itself. It can also be a great deal more painful. After the menopause, breasts normally stop being painful. If the sensations do continue then you should seek advice.

> *For about eight days in each month my breasts would become full and incredibly tender. I couldn't bear them to be touched, and some nights I would have to sleep on my back. Oddly enough it didn't seem to be linked to my periods and it was only when I finally went to a breast clinic that I got some reassurance.*

What you can do

Any unusual sensations or changes around the breast should be investigated if only to reassure you that there is nothing wrong. Over five million women a year experience breast pain, known as mastalgia, and yet in the vast majority of cases there is nothing seriously wrong. Part of the problem with breast pain is the anxiety it arouses, but it may reassure you to know that there is rarely any pain of this kind associated with breast cancer.

Your doctor may ask you to keep a diary over three months of when the pain occurs, to establish whether it is cyclical (linked to your menstrual cycle) or non-cyclical. If it is cyclical and very painful you may be offered evening primrose oil. Taken in a daily dose of 3g, this is effective in many cases. You may be able to get this on prescription, but check the prices because it can sometimes be cheaper to buy these supplements over the counter. Look carefully at the type of evening primrose oil and make sure it is the correct strength – this also applies to all other supplements you may want to take.

If you find no relief from this, then there are a couple of drugs – Danazol and Bromocriptine – that may be offered as alternative treatments. Both have some side-effects, such as weight gain, headaches and nausea. Tamoxifen, a drug used for treating breast cancer, can also be prescribed in short courses and under careful supervision.

However, you may want to try some self-help measures, such as checking that the bra you wear fits properly and is offering the right support. Some women find that wearing a comfortable bra at night to support the breasts can help too. You can also look at your diet, as some research suggests there may be a connection between painful, sore breasts and fluid retention, too much caffeine and diets that are high in fat.

If the breast pain is not linked to your period (i.e. it is non-cyclical), it may be that the pain is not coming from the breast at all but from areas around it – the ribs and muscles under the breast are common areas. Examination will discover the location, and pain-killers such as ibuprofen will usually be effective.

Breast lumps
The most reassuring thing about breast lumps is that the vast majority are not cancerous. Many women can feel lumps in their breasts, and these are usually easier to feel just before a period. If you examine your breasts fairly regularly preferably at around the same time of the month you will know their usual feel, so if a new lump appears you should spot it early on. The instructions on page 58 show you how to examine your breasts.

During the menopause, breast cysts are quite common because they appear as breast tissue ages. They are recognizable as smooth lumps that tend to move slightly as you touch them. A large cyst is easy to see, while you may just locate the smaller ones with the pads of your fingers. They can also be painful. If you find a lump in your breast, the first investigation will usually be mammography (a breast X-ray) or ultrasound. Once the cyst has been identified, the doctor will insert a very fine needle into it to extract the fluid. Usually this makes the cyst disappear, so no further treatment is needed. If the fluid from the cyst is blood-stained then it will be sent for tests, but in other cases, when the fluid is yellowish, no further tests are carried out. A cyst does not mean you will develop breast cancer, and most women who develop a cyst will only have the one. Some women will have several during their lifetime; in this case, although there is a slightly increased risk of cancer, it is not a significant one.

Nipple changes

The nipples do alter slightly as a woman ages – they may pull in and there may be a creamy discharge. In most cases there will be nothing to worry about. Some discharge from the nipple can occur as a result of an infection of the ducts, which is easy to treat, but any change in the nipples should always be checked by your doctor. You are likely to be sent for a mammogram just to make sure that none of the changes is due to cancer. Any bleeding from the nipple should be reported to the doctor as soon as possible.

Breast cancer

Your risk of developing breast cancer does increase as you get older, but the majority of lumps found are still more likely to be benign.

Some women are at higher risk than others: if you fall into any of the following groups, make sure that you attend for regular screening, and if you do find a lump or a change in breast or nipple shape see your doctor without any delay.

You are at higher risk of breast cancer if the following circumstances apply to you:

- *Family history* Some women have inherited a gene which makes them more likely to develop breast cancer. Your risk is higher if a close family member has had breast cancer (or cancer of the ovaries, colon or prostate) while under the age of 50, or if several family members have or have had breast cancer. Research in this area is progressing fast and several of the breast cancer genes have been identified. In some places, testing for abnormal genes is already available.
- *Age* The older you are, the greater the chances of breast cancer. The risk approximately doubles every ten years.
- *Late maternity* A first pregnancy after the age of 30 or never having children puts you at increased risk.
- *HRT* You are at a slightly increased risk if you take HRT for more than ten years.
- *Lifestyle* If you drink heavily or are very overweight and if your diet is high in fats you may be at increased risk. A link between smoking and breast cancer has not been proved, but there is

increasing evidence to show that eating a healthy, balanced diet can increase your immunity to breast cancer.

- *Late natural menopause* If you are still having regular periods after the age of 52, you are at higher risk of breast and uterine cancer.

Erratic periods

A change in your periods is often the first sign that you are entering the peri-menopause. You may be one of the very small number of women who find that their periods stop from one month to the next and never start again. This is unusual, and if it is due to oestrogen levels falling sharply you may experience quite severe symptoms such as hot flushes. On the other hand, for some women the menopause occurs almost as a single event with very few additional symptoms.

For most women, however, the ending of periods is quite a gradual process, with periods becoming lighter and shorter until eventually they cease altogether. There may be some irregularity as well, but if periods tail off in this way the chances are that you will experience fewer menopausal symptoms. In other cases your periods may vary tremendously.

Irregular and unpredictable periods can be very irritating to live with. One month you may bleed very heavily, the next month there will be practically nothing at all. A few weeks later you may get an 'ordinary' period but it may last for nearly a fortnight or just for a day or two. Gaps between periods may vary from a couple of weeks to several months.

Some women experience 'flooding' – occasional very heavy bleeds which can be very embarrassing if they occur in the wrong place at the wrong time. It's always a good idea to see the doctor about these, as they may be due to an underlying cause such as polyps, fibroids or endometriosis.

Bleeding after periods have been absent for more than six months should be discussed with your doctor.

What you can do

Once you've confirmed that there is nothing radically wrong, erratic periods should be regarded as simply part of the approaching menopause. However, if your periods are heavier than usual or very frequent, or if you are experiencing flooding, it makes sense to ask for a blood test to make sure that you are not anaemic. If you are, then your doctor will prescribe iron tablets, and you can help yourself by eating plenty of iron-rich foods such as wheat, accompanied by vitamin C to help the iron to be properly absorbed.

Signs of ageing

It's one of the first outward signs of the menopause – your skin condition begins to change. More wrinkles appear on your face and neck, brown spots may appear on your hands, your skin may also become more sensitive and you may find your normal moisturizer or make-up produces an allergic reaction.

You will need to take extra care in the sun. Over 30,000 people a year get skin cancer in Britain, and the best way to protect yourself is to stop sunbathing and use a moisturizer with an SPF (sun protection factor) of at least 15 on your face and lips all year round.

When you can't avoid being in the sun, use a sunscreen with SPF 15 on all exposed parts of the body, but get into the habit of covering up – wear a hat, a T-shirt, lightweight long skirts or trousers. Many items of clothing for outdoor use, such as hats, T-shirts, trousers and long-sleeved tops, are now available in a weave that can actually keep out some of the sun's rays, so they are worth considering if, for instance, you are planning a long-distance walk.

Some forms of skin cancer are linked to a build-up of exposure to the sun, so keep an eye on any existing moles and see your doctor as soon as possible if you notice any changes in shape, colour, size or any bleeding, as most cancers respond very well to treatment in the early stages.

You may also notice other skin changes. You may develop dark rings under your eyes or tiny broken veins on the face and legs; unwanted hair may begin to sprout around the chin and upper lip; gums may start to cause problems by receding or regularly becoming infected; and your hair will feel thinner and be less glossy. When you brush or comb it, a lot may seem to be falling out. You will find that you put on weight as the metabolism slows down – there's no harm in gaining a few extra pounds and you should be able to keep weight gain under control by sensible eating and regular exercise.

All these changes are due to your hormones. Lower levels of oestrogen have a knock-on effect on supplies of collagen, making the skin thinner and less resilient. Underneath the skin, nerve endings are ageing, less blood is flowing through and muscles are losing tone. One of the most uncomfortable problems in this area is itching and irritation of the skin. Quite a number of women experience formication – a tingling feeling that really does feel as if ants are crawling across the skin.

What you can do

Although most women come to terms with the fact that they are gradually gaining a few more wrinkles and that those already there are deeper, it is becoming much more acceptable to use various treatments such as collagen injections, skin peeling and laser treatments to rejuvenate the face, as women in the fifties age group are healthier, more active and younger in outlook than any previous generation. There are also surgical techniques that can adjust, lift, smooth and tuck almost every part of your body.

However, because it is thinner, your skin does need protection, so a daily moisturizer is essential, and preferably one that already contains a sunscreen. When you cleanse the skin, do so gently – try not to drag at the skin, especially the very delicate skin under the eyes.

Although many of the physical symptoms and changes that take place during the menopause can be very upsetting and disturbing, the vast majority are not life-threatening. That is not to underestimate their importance. Any woman who is in a state of utter exhaustion following months of broken nights due to night sweats, or who has had to try to keep a cool head during important meetings while hot flushes sweep over her, has a right to feel that her life is being thoroughly disturbed – and to feel depressed about it.

No one really knows why some women suffer more than others – whether it is due to an attitude of mind, to stress, to genetics – but understanding why these changes are occurring and knowing that, in most cases, a choice of treatments to relieve the symptoms is available, can make a difference to the way you handle your life.

3

What's happening to your mind?

There's no doubt that the menopause can often be a very turbulent time. Falling oestrogen levels affect you not only physically but emotionally and mentally too.

Among the most commonly reported conditions are depression, loss of concentration, memory problems, panic attacks, anxiety and mood swings. It doesn't seem to matter who you are. You can be a high-powered career woman or a mother of six who has never gone out to work; you can be married, divorced or single, have young or grown-up children or no children at all. You can still experience the same feelings, a similar upheaval.

Many women are led to believe that emotional symptoms at this time are entirely due to the menopause, but although fluctuating hormone levels do play a part in many cases – and produce symptoms that are very similar to PMS (pre-menstrual syndrome) – this may not be the whole story. The danger of attributing these changes simply to the menopause is that they may not be treated appropriately or may even be left untreated altogether.

Knowing what to expect and realizing that it happens to a lot of other women can help reduce your own levels of stress and anxiety. It also helps to understand that many menopausal symptoms are short-lived and that the physical ones can often be treated very successfully.

In the countries where little is made of either the physical or emotional symptoms of the menopause, and where this stage is almost celebrated as a rite of passage, women often barely experience them. Some studies have reported that women who view this time as natural and look to the future with confidence have fewer emotional symptoms such as depression and problems over concentration. However, there are plenty of women who enter the menopause in a calm frame of mind and are completely bowled over by the severity of their symptoms.

I just didn't recognize myself. From being a highly organized, efficient person I became this complete scatterbrain. It took a tremendous effort to cover up my loss of concentration and the forgetfulness. I developed all sorts of strategies to cope on a daily basis in the office. I had lists and Post-it notes all over my desk

31

and I lived in fear of being found out. I think it drained me – in the evenings and at weekends, times I'd always enjoyed, I simply collapsed and would spend a lot of time dozing.

The worst thing of all for me were the mood swings. I became very touchy, very irritable, flying off the handle at the least little thing. The next minute I'd be in floods of tears at a sad item on the television news.

In many cases, medical treatments may well be the answer, but before you make this decision it makes sense to analyse exactly what is going on in your life apart from the menopause, to see if this can give a clue to some of your changes of mood or character.

If you are now in your forties and fifties you may well be starting to reassess your life. If you had your children in your twenties and thirties, they will now be more or less grown up. Some will be teenagers, demanding even more of your time and energy than you might have expected as you worry about exams, drugs, discipline, their future. There may well be areas of conflict over their friends, staying out late, untidiness, school work.

Although some parents find the teenage years rewarding as they become good friends with their offspring, for others it comes as a shock when the adorable and adored child suddenly changes into an apparently uncontrollable monster. Teenagers are also going through an hormonal upheaval, and with similar hormones involved there are plenty of opportunities for a clash of wills and temperaments.

If your children are that bit older they may be leaving home, travelling, studying, finding their first job, marrying or starting a family. The 'empty nest syndrome' is well recognized as a disconcerting time for both parents, but for mothers in particular. On the one hand you rejoice that your main parenting has been successfully completed and the fledgling is about to leave the nest, but at the same time you worry about what will happen to them in the big wide world. Have you passed on the right lessons? Will they remember all your good and sensible advice while they are away? Thinking back to your own youth you probably know the answer to that!

The marriage of their children and becoming a grandparent are two more big milestones for women at this time. As your child sets off on his/her new life journey, new links are forged and some may be broken. Priorities change as the most important person in your child's life is someone else. From now on, for the relationship to be successful, it's important for loyalties to change – clinging at this stage or making your child feel guilty for putting their partner's needs first, rather than yours, can cause unnecessary tension and risks driving you apart.

Once grandchildren come on the scene there is a really big change. Grandchildren represent the future, and suddenly it may feel as if you have taken a step back. It reinforces the reality of the years ahead and your place in the generations.

For more and more women, the menopause falls closer to their years of child-bearing as they choose to delay the start of a family in order to establish a career. You may perhaps have much higher expectations of marriage and partnerships, and this can often mean that you haven't begun to think about having children until your mid to late thirties. It's no longer unusual to have a first child in your forties, or to add to an existing family in those years. Divorce can also often result in a second family later in life. This can all be very confusing as, on the one hand, you have the living evidence of your fertility in front of you while, on the other, your body is beginning to give very different messages. If you have tried unsuccessfully to have children or have not yet made the decision, the first symptoms of the menopause will come as confirmation that time is indeed running out.

Another, increasingly large, group of women find that the years of the menopause may coincide with having to take responsibility for elderly parents and relatives. Just when you felt that your life was becoming easier, with fewer responsibilities and at last the time to do some of the things you want, so new commitments, often quite distressing and stressful ones, may arise.

For single women and those with careers, this may be the time for a rethink. Readjustments need to be made or are sometimes forced on you. If you have worked hard for much of your adult life, you may be starting to wonder whether it is all worth it, whether you need to stand back and take a good hard look at your working life.

Although there has been a change in attitude towards women at work, the glass ceiling that prevents so many from reaching their full potential still exists, and although you might be able to protest at overt sexual discrimination, it is often so subtly done that you have little or no ammunition to fight your corner. At the same time, younger women and men are often being promoted to work alongside or above you.

You may also feel particularly sensitive at work about possibly obvious menopause symptoms such as hot flushes being noticed and remarked upon – invariably without much understanding and usually behind your back. It's just another area of stress to cope with.

Despite changes and the realization that mature workers have a great deal to offer, women are no more secure than men when redundancy threatens. An employer will often look at the balance sheet first, and an older worker is always more expensive than a newly qualified younger person.

From all this you can see that plenty of things are likely to be happening in your life at this time. Very often you may be having to juggle a whole range of different roles and as a result may be under considerable stress. That is why establishing cause and effect of some of the emotional symptoms you may feel is not as cut and dried as it might be.

So what are the most common symptoms at this time – and what can be done about them?

Depression

It's not at all unusual for a women to report that she is feeling depressed at this stage in her life; treatment will depend on how acute the depression is and its possible causes. As well as all the life changes mentioned above, some women do find it hard to come to terms with actually being menopausal, never mind any of the symptoms, so some degree of depression is not surprising. Some research has shown that a woman who finds it hard to come to terms with being menopausal has a higher chance of experiencing some emotional repercussions.

At the mildest level, depression will show itself as a general lack of interest and enthusiasm. It is as if you are seeing life through a thin grey curtain – you can still see everything, but it is vague and slightly blurred, the colours are washed out, and sounds are muted or provoke little response. There is a sense of being weighed down and exhausted. Many everyday things become an effort, and it may take you longer to complete tasks you previously found quite simple – and as for taking on anything more complex, forget it.

Depression is often accompanied by disturbed sleep. You may find you fall asleep quickly but wake a few hours later and find it impossible to drop off again; you may find it hard to go to sleep in the first place or you may wake in the early hours of the morning. The quality of your sleep can also be affected so that even if you do sleep reasonably well, you wake unrefreshed.

You may delay seeing the doctor, but if and when you do see her, try and book a longer appointment so that she can make a better assessment of your condition and what treatment, if any, might be appropriate.

However, you should certainly see your doctor if you have three or more of the following symptoms of depression and they have lasted for longer than two weeks:

- a change in your sleeping patterns – either broken sleep, insomnia or excessive sleepiness;
- feeling very weary, totally lacking in energy;
- feeling very sad and tearful;
- lack of interest in sex;
- feeling restless, jumpy;
- feeling very low about yourself and your abilities;
- finding it hard to concentrate, focus on or enjoy anything.

If you start to have thoughts of suicide or death or consider attempting suicide, you should see your doctor or seek help without delay.

What can be done

The first priority is to try to establish the cause of your depression. Because the parts of the brain that influence some of your positive emotions, such as feelings of stability and well-being, are affected by a lack of oestrogen, some experts believe that for some women, hormone replacement treatment (HRT) may be very helpful. If some of the symptoms of depression appear to you to be specifically due to the menopause, then increasing levels of oestrogen could be the answer. For instance, if night sweats are keeping you awake and making you feel exhausted and generally low during the day, then some treatment, whether with conventional medicine or complementary therapies, will improve your sleep and help you to cope better.

However, if your life is stressful in other ways at the moment or if you are finding it hard to come to terms with the changes that are taking place in your body, this could well be a trigger for a depressive episode that has less to do with the physiological changes of the menopause and your lower oestrogen levels.

If you and your doctor discuss this and feel that it may be the case, your doctor may suggest you see a counsellor, a psychologist or psychiatrist in order to talk through and try to resolve some of the things that are worrying you. Alternatively, she may suggest you take a course of anti-depressants to boost the level of serotonin in the brain, which is depleted by depression, particularly if it has been going on for some time. Treatment would normally be prescribed for three to six months.

What you can do

- Above all, you need to give yourself time and space. It's hard, when you are feeling low, even to summon up the energy to do the things that you might enjoy, but it is worth trying to find the time to take a walk in the country, spend time with a close friend, have a long, warm bath or treat yourself to an aromatherapy massage.

- Try to share some of your feelings, either with your partner or with close friends; talking can often relieve some of the tension and sadness.

- There may be a self-help group in your area which you could join. People often report that it helps them to feel less isolated knowing there are others experiencing similar feelings.

- Take regular exercise. Although you may feel tired, 20 minutes of physical activity three or more times a week can help to lift your mood as exercise releases endorphins, the body's natural anti-depressants, which can give you a mood boost that lasts for several hours. Exercise also makes you feel good about yourself and what you can achieve, and it is increasingly 'prescribed' by doctors as a way to treat depression, whether on its own or alongside other forms of treatment (see Chapter 5).

- If your life is very stressful and you often feel you are being pulled in several directions at once by the demands made on you, include regular relaxation or meditation, or gentle exercise such as yoga or T'ai chi in your daily routine. Even snatching ten minutes each day to sit still and silent can be helpful.

- Cut down on alcohol and smoking – neither are particularly good for you, and alcohol in excess of more than a couple of glasses won't improve sleep or lift your mood.

- Watch what you eat – choose foods that have plenty of B vitamins (such as meat, especially the juices, which you can use in gravy); dairy products such as cheese, yoghurt, milk; wholegrain cereals and brown rice; green vegetables, especially broccoli and spinach; fruits, especially bananas and dried apricots, figs or dates.

- Herbal remedies such as St John's Wort (hypericum) seem to work well with mild depression. In one study, people (not just women) taking it were compared with those on one of the newer anti-depressants, and the results showed a better outcome for those on the herbal preparation. In Germany, where it is very commonly prescribed to treat depression, a study of menopausal women showed that 80 per cent felt it helped relieve their depression, and 60 per cent of those who took part reported that it had improved their libido following a 12-week course. However, it is now known that hypericum can interact with other drugs, including anti-coagulants such as Warfarin and immunosuppressants. You should discuss this with your doctor.

- Another herbal remedy worth considering is wild yam. It contains disogenin, which seems able to help balance oestrogen levels in the body. In the laboratory, oestrogen and progesterone can be synthesized from wild yam, but the wild yam you buy in most health stories and pharmacies will not do this.
- Some women find that a supplement containing zinc and magnesium can help to lift their mood. Your diet can provide good amounts of these minerals. Seeds are good sources of zinc, while magnesium is found in root vegetables and green vegetables such as cabbage.

For more about natural remedies see Chapter 7.

Insomnia

Some research with menopausal women has shown that their quality of sleep is different, with far less deep sleep than other people. Less rapid eye movement (REM) sleep means that you wake less refreshed. However, various types of insomnia, when you either have difficulty getting to sleep or wake up several times in the night or in the early hours, frequently accompany depression. Poor sleep can also be the result of frequent night sweats, anxiety and stress.

You will probably know better than anyone else what may be causing your insomnia. Often it cannot be treated on its own because it is so closely linked to another symptom. In other cases the insomnia may be due to a variety of quite specific causes, and you may need to address or treat them one by one.

What you can do

If you suffer from a physical symptom such as night sweats then you will need to deal with this first. If you are being woken several times a night every night with night sweats or aching limbs, it is hardly surprising that you will begin to feel that everything is getting on top of you.

Follow the suggestions in Chapter 2 to deal with night sweats and make sure you are comfortable in bed.

If your life is very fraught at the moment then this type of stress can easily manifest itself as insomnia. You may not wake up and worry about the next day, but you could well have disturbed nights.

Lack of sleep or poor sleep has a tremendous impact on the way you function and how you cope, so it is worth making an effort to resolve the problem. In many cases this can be achieved without resorting to sleeping pills, although you may find that a short course can help re-establish a very disrupted sleep pattern that has been going on for years.

Anxiety and panic attacks

Many women do feel anxious and panicky at the menopause, and these feelings may be linked in with an underlying depression. If you are experiencing a loss of confidence about yourself, your looks, your ability to cope or what lies ahead, it can often result in anxiety, particularly in certain situations.

It is also possible that you have been under stress for some time and that the additional symptoms of the menopause – the possible embarrassment of hot flushes, headaches, loss of libido – just make everything harder to handle.

You may be finding that you have started to worry a lot more. The trouble is that once you start thinking this way it is hard to stop. You may often feel uncomfortable in social situations, concerned that you may say the wrong thing or not be wearing the right clothes. You will perhaps begin to make excuses to avoid situations that you feel may emphasize your lack of confidence. If your feelings of anxiety remain untreated, they may develop into a form of agoraphobia and make it almost impossible for you to go out. The feelings of panic that can be associated with this anxiety are also quite common – you may feel your heart beating faster, break out into a sweat (as opposed to a hot flush) and feel breathless, dizzy or faint.

What you can do

You should try and talk to your doctor about what you are feeling. If your anxiety is linked to menopausal symptoms such as severe hot flushes or night sweats, she may suggest hormone replacement as a possible solution. Some women have found that increasing their levels of oestrogen can reduce feelings of anxiety and give them some additional confidence.

If you are looking for your own solutions, you will find that many of those suggested for depression (above) can be helpful. It's particularly useful to be able to share these often inexplicable feelings of anxiety with other people in a similar situation, so if there is a self-help group in your area you might consider joining.

As with so many psychological symptoms at the time of the menopause, it is always worth spending time looking for what is contributing to your feelings of anxiety. Maybe you have money worries, stress at work, concerns about your family or a feeling that your relationship with your partner is shaky. Until you have begun to sort out these problem areas, it will be hard to reduce the feelings of anxiety and panic.

Once you have begun to deal with underlying problems, you can introduce relaxation and calming techniques into your life that will help you to cope better with your anxiety.

Visualization

Some women have found that visualization techniques work really well for them. You need to take time to sit in a quiet place where you are not going to be disturbed. Make yourself comfortable in a chair or on the floor, breathe evenly and, with your eyes closed, conjure up an image of something or somewhere that gives you pleasure and where you feel relaxed and at ease – maybe a beach, a country meadow, a mountain stream. If you find this hard initially, maybe you can find a drawing or photograph to look at. While you visualize, you try to think positively about yourself and your situation. Find phrases that you can repeat to yourself that will encourage you to create positive thoughts, such as, 'I am a very capable and loving person.'

If the anxiety or panic attacks are frequent then you could benefit from cognitive behavioural therapy, which aims to retrain you to face your fears and phobias little by little, so that eventually you learn to control these feelings.

Mood swings

These take many women by surprise by their violence and unpredictability – although if you have experienced pre-menstrual tension you will recognize the scenario.

> *I just couldn't recognize myself. One minute I'd be this perfectly rational, pleasant person, and the next I'd either be yelling and screaming or in floods of tears. It was usually sparked off by something quite minor. I don't know how my partner and children put up with me.*

Although not all doctors agree that these changes in mood can be laid at the door of our hormones, mood swings do seem to be very much part of the hormonal changes that are taking place – the peaks and troughs of oestrogen as it surges from low to high levels. If you are experiencing quite strong symptoms and they are occurring without warning, this can be very unsettling and result in frequent changes of mood from high to low, from relaxed to irritable. It may also be that the way you feel about the menopause has an effect on your mood. If you feel angry about the changes that are taking place, you are more likely to respond irrationally.

The most common mood problems revolve around anger and frustration. You may begin to find it almost unbearable to be stuck in a traffic jam or to have to queue for tickets or at the check-out. You may also find that you become very blinkered about yourself – insisting on doing things that others know will exhaust you or aren't really necessary. When others gently try to point this out, the balloon goes up again. Much of this is linked to stress and also perhaps to feelings of insecurity about your own abilities.

Part of this approach also cuts out your awareness of other people and their needs, or even what they might have to contribute.

What you can do

- It is time to stand back and let go now and then – not because you are giving up but because you have the confidence to take a back seat.
- Try not to take on too much – conserve your energies for the things that really matter. Each day, make a list of what has to be done and feel pleased with yourself if you can cross off three or four of the more important ones.
- If you are in a traffic jam or check-out queue, try to switch off from the fact that you are being kept waiting. Take slow deep breaths, talk to the person next to you. If you are in a car, play a story tape; if you are waiting in a queue always have something to read – a newspaper, a book. It's amazing how much more quickly the time goes when you give your mind something else to think about.
- Always allow yourself plenty of time to get anywhere – if you arrive early then think of it as time gained.
- Stand outside yourself occasionally and listen to what others have to say about you, about themselves.
- Next time you feel yourself beginning to get angry about something, pause for a moment to ask yourself if there is anything

you can do to change the situation. In most cases you will find it is quite out of your control and that the way to cope with other people is to change your attitude towards them.

- Rather than nagging others to change, to do things your way, to conform to your rules or ways of behaviour, realize that change will only come if *they* want it, not because you insist on it or even suggest it. Your solution, for your own peace of mind, is to learn the art of the shrug when something begins to annoy you and you can feel yourself coming up to the boil, shrug your shoulders, either physically or mentally, and say to yourself, 'So what? There's nothing I can do to alter this. I shall ignore it.'

Memory loss

A huge number of menopausal and peri-menopausal women suffer from forgetfulness, find it hard to concentrate or experience moments of confusion. Often these lapses seem pretty trivial. Locking the car keys in the car, forgetting items of shopping or making a list and leaving it at home, suddenly having to think about how to get somewhere for a journey you've done many times, forgetting to pass on an important message, searching for words, going into a room and forgetting what you are there for – the list is endless.

If you have previously been fairly well organized it can be very worrying, so it's not surprising that you may begin to wonder whether you are losing your mind, going mad or possibly experiencing early symptoms of dementia.

It's important to remember the other things that may be going on at the moment, and the other possible reasons for these episodes of forgetfulness. For instance, if you are suffering from insomnia, you need to know that fatigue often leads to memory lapses. It is also recognized that depression and, in particular, stress can make it harder to concentrate.

There are oestrogen receptors in the brain which, as oestrogen levels drop, may have a role to play. More recent research is beginning to uncover a possible link between Alzheimer's Disease and Parkinson's Disease and the free radicals that can destroy tissue. Antioxidants can offer protection against free radicals by mopping them up and these are found in many fresh foods. However, it is now known that oestrogen is also an antioxidant, which, given its presence in the brain, may therefore have a role to play in protecting brain tissue against free radical damage, and may perhaps lower the risk of diseases such as Alzheimer's developing.

Other research has produced results showing that post-menopausal women on hormone replacement therapy performed better in tests on short-term visual memory than those not on HRT. However, a lot more research will be needed before HRT can be prescribed to improve memory and perhaps protect against Alzheimer's.

What you can do

Self-help is one of the best solutions if you are finding your memory is letting you down. As with the body, the key words are 'use it or lose it'. In order to function well, the brain needs exercise. Each day give it a good stretch – a crossword or a puzzle to solve, a short poem or speech to learn.

Develop strategies to help you deal with your slightly less reliable memory. Be as organized as possible, and always put things in the same place – keys on a hook, shopping lists on a noticeboard, appointments on a large, visible diary.

Make a point of writing everything down it makes things much easier to remember once you have seen them in writing. When you've met some new people, try and write down their names as soon as you get in and if you have difficulty putting a name to a face, think of a distinguishing feature to jog the memory next time you meet.

Make lists a part of your life, but don't let them rule you. Have a board in the kitchen for shopping: as soon as you think of something that's needed next time you go shopping, write it on the list where it is visible. Do the same for appointments.

The brain needs to be stimulated and challenged and not allowed to get into a rut. This is the time to take on a new challenge: try something you've always wanted to do but never had the time or inclination to attempt, like learning a new language, taking up pottery or photography, embarking on an Open University degree, learning to play a musical instrument or joining a choir. Meeting new people is always stimulating, whether through voluntary work, a new hobby or interest or on holiday.

The way you look

Some women find the visible signs of ageing quite easy to come to terms with. They may notice the extra wrinkles on their face, a slight sagging round the neck and a thickening of the waist, and simply take it all on board. But for others it is extremely distressing, and in a society where the emphasis is still very much on youth, despite the fact that the over fifties are in the majority, the need to do something about it is very strong.

Cosmetic surgery

The days when the facelift was effectively the only option are in the past. Women today have more choices – skin-peeling, laser treatments, injections. However, these treatments are surgical, so before you agree to anything you should be sure that the person performing it is properly qualified, with full insurance, and that you feel at ease and know everything you need to know about the procedure, including any risks, the cost, pain relief and recovery time. Ideally, get everything put in writing. Your GP may know a consultant plastic surgeon who specializes in cosmetic surgery, or should be able to get you a list of qualified people. Be very wary of clinics advertising in glossy magazines. Take time to make a decision.

> *I thought long and hard about it, but in my job I was constantly coming into contact with women in their mid to late thirties who looked so good. I felt more and more unconfident about my appearance. In the end cosmetic surgery was the only solution. It made a tremendous difference, not just to my looks but to the way I felt about myself.*

Other options

If you don't want to submit to such drastic procedures there are other options. Collagen injections fill out lines and wrinkles, and a variety of non-surgical treatments which use electrical tools to stimulate the skin claim to make a difference. Although some women report that their skin feels and looks firmer, the change tends to last only as long as the treatments continue, so it can work out quite expensive.

A salon facial may not take away all your wrinkles but your skin will probably look brighter, and it's a good way of ensuring that you lie still and relax for an hour or so. Don't have a facial more than once every couple of months as the treatment may irritate the skin. Some beauty therapists advise older women to avoid steaming to open the pores as this can result in broken capillaries. If your skin is or has become very sensitive, it may also be a good idea to test the products used beforehand to make sure they are suitable. If a mask is going to be used, make sure it is not too drying for your skin – most skins at this age need moisturizing.

Facial hair is extremely embarrassing for many women at the menopause. Individual hairs can be removed at home with a good pair of tweezers or in a salon with electrolysis – you will need several treatments to ensure all hair has been removed. Some women use wax or depilatories, and laser hair removal is now more common, although no one is yet sure of the possible long-term effects. If you prefer not to remove the hair, bleaching is an option.

Good make-up, well applied, can make a tremendous difference. Most women use the same make-up in their fifties that they used in their twenties. One way round this is to have a free make-up session in a department store – that way you'll learn about new products and what works for you. The basic rule is: the more wrinkles you have, the less make-up, especially foundation, you will need. A heavy foundation will not cover up wrinkles and lines – all it does is sink into them and make them more obvious. You may find now that you only need to apply a foundation in certain areas, such as on either side of the nose, on shadows under the eyes and on the eyelids. Apply lightly and blend well; choosing exactly the right colour for your skin makes this a lot easier. You may feel more comfortable not using foundation but just applying some blusher to cheek-bones over a tinted moisturizer.

Take a look at your hair – there is no need to have short hair after the age of 40, but long hair especially does need to be kept in good condition and trimmed regularly. If your hair is thinning then a short haircut can make the most of what you've got. Make use of the products on the market to give your thinning hair more volume, and have a fringe if your forehead is very lined and you want to hide it.

If you want to cover up the grey, in the early stages a rinse or a semi-permanent colourant usually works well. If you are grey all over and don't want to be, then a permanent colouring treatment will be needed, although roots will have to be touched up every four to six weeks. Choose a colour that complements your skin and remember that light colours will make thinning hair look thinner. Some women find it easier to go for high or lowlights which blend in other colours with the grey; this makes it easier to go grey all over if and when you choose to and means you don't have to touch up the roots.

Healthy, shiny hair is very dependent on what goes on inside, so eating well can make all the difference.

4

Medical complaints

The symptoms that you experience as you go through the menopause tend not to last for long. However, it is now recognized that the changes taking place in your body at this time do increase your chances of experiencing some health problems. In some cases your genetic make-up will increase your risk, but in many instances taking care of yourself from now on can do a great deal to help you avoid these complications.

Osteoporosis

This is now the most common health problem for women in later life. One in three women will suffer from it by the age of 80. Osteoporosis is a disorder in which our bones become thinner and less dense as we age, increasing the chances of fracture. Men suffer from osteoporosis too, although less commonly.

Healthy bones are in a continuous state of repair and renewal, with old bone being broken down and replaced thanks to the activity of special cells called osteoclasts, which destroy the old bone, and osteoblasts, which create new bone. Their function is controlled by several different hormones, including oestrogen. Oestrogen also plays a part in ensuring that the bones absorb calcium well in order to remain strong.

For women, bone loss starts from the age of about 40. At first this is gradual, but during the menopause the falling oestrogen levels speed up the whole process. Bone loss means that the inside structure of the bone changes: holes appear, making the bone less dense, and if no action is taken quite a minor fall can cause a fracture.

The problem with osteoporosis is that there are no symptoms at all until the disease is well advanced. Often the first signs of bone-thinning are when there is a fracture. The most common fractures occur in the wrists, ankles, hips, spine and collar-bone, and most fractures occur in much older women – over the age of 65. The older you are, the more chance there is of a fracture seriously affecting your independence. A fracture late in life can be very painful and recovery is slow. You can end up housebound and unable to care for yourself. Osteoporosis is also life-threatening to older women; many elderly women who suffer a hip fracture die within six months from other health problems or complications, because the initial fall may be a reflection of their frailty and overall state of health.

On the positive side, if changes in bone density are detected in the early stages, treatments have now been developed to halt bone loss or at least slow it down. Increasingly, thanks to the development of new drugs, bone can be strengthened.

There is no established screening programme for osteoporosis in the UK, but groups of people at high risk have been identified. If you fall into any of the following groups then you should request a bone density scan through your GP. Evidence shows that identifying people at highest risk and treating them can halve their risk of developing osteoporosis.

You may be at higher risk of developing osteoporosis if you

- have had a hysterectomy before the age of the menopause involving removal of your ovaries, or even a premature menopause with ovarian conservation;
- are a heavy smoker;
- regularly take steroid tablets such as prednisolone for conditions such as arthritis or asthma;
- have had an early menopause, not caused by surgery (before the age of 45);
- have suffered from prolonged amenorrhoea (lack of periods) before the menopause;
- did little or no exercise in your teens and twenties;
- have a past history of fractures;
- have lost height;
- have had bowel disease or surgery.

Evidence also shows that fair-skinned, small, slender people are at higher risk, as are those whose parents suffered from osteoporosis, especially if there has been a history of hip fractures on your mother's side.

Screening

Measuring bone mass is the best way to identify osteoporosis before a fracture occurs. The most widely used method is DEXA (dual energy X-ray absorptiometry). This machine takes measurements of bone density in your spine, hips and wrist. The procedure is totally painless and takes around 15 minutes – although newer machines can perform the same task much more quickly. You lie on a bed, fully clothed and with a large foam block under your thighs to keep your back straight. The scanning machine at your side passes along your body. If your doctor feels that you fall within the high-risk group for osteoporosis, she may request a scan to confirm the diagnosis. Shockingly, many areas of the UK still do not have GP access to the DEXA machines needed for this simple screening.

If you have signs of spinal fracture such as back pain and height loss due to osteoporosis, then the doctor may request an X-ray instead.

Prevention

There are several ways in which both those at risk and those with reasonable bone density at the menopause can at least slow down the loss in bone mass and hopefully prevent fractures occurring later in their lives.

Calcium

Nearly all the calcium we have is deposited in our bones. This mineral is a vital way to prevent bone loss so it's important to have an adequate intake of calcium. The suggested amount is 1200mg a day during the menopause and 1400mg a day post-menopause. A pint of milk contains about 750mg, and there is a little more calcium in skimmed milk that in semi-skimmed or full cream; 100g of cheddar cheese contains 800mg. Although dairy produce is a good source, calcium is also easily available from fish, especially the bones of tinned sardines, tinned salmon and tinned pilchards. If you find it hard to have enough calcium from your diet then you may want to take a calcium supplement. Some foods, such as spinach, wholewheat cereals, zinc supplements, coffee, alcohol and antacids to treat indigestion, can hinder the absorption of calcium, as do fizzy cola drinks, so take supplements at a different time. Lack of vitamin D, which is made by the skin absorbing sunlight, can also cause bone loss. This is far more likely to be a problem among older women who may not go out much. However, taken as a supplement with calcium, vitamin D enhances the way calcium is absorbed.

Exercise

Weight-bearing exercise – jogging or brisk walking two or three times a week – can make a real difference to bone density, especially pre-menopause. But it is never too late to start to reduce the effects of osteoporosis. (For further advice on all forms of exercise see Chapter 5.)

Drugs

The main drugs currently used to help prevent osteoporosis are hormone replacement therapy (HRT), bisphosphonates such as alendronate and Risedronate, which are also used to treat the condition, and SERMs, a new generation of hormone therapy (see below).

Hormone replacement therapy

For most women at high risk of osteoporosis, HRT has tended to be the first choice because it has been shown to prevent further bone loss and increase bone density, both during and after the menopause. HRT can be started at any time after the menopause to treat osteoporosis, but if you are still peri-menopausal, having irregular periods and there is a chance of pregnancy you will be advised to use some form of contraception along with HRT. At the moment it is still not clear whether the beneficial effects of HRT on bone mass can be sustained once treatment ceases, so most women on HRT for osteoporosis will be advised to stay on it for between five and ten years, after which time treatment will be reviewed. As new, non-hormonal treatments are developed, women will be able to choose these after the menopause. (For more about HRT see Chapter 6.)

Bisphosphonates

Bisphosphonates work by preventing the osteoclasts from destroying bone. The main types used at the moment are etidronate, which is prescribed as Didronel PMO, and alendronate, prescribed as Fosamax and Risedronate (Actonel). The etidronate is taken as a pill once a day for two weeks, followed by 76 days of calcium supplements. Some women experience side-effects such as nausea from etidronate. Fosamax and Actonel are taken as daily tablets.

The bisphosphonates may cause severe indigestion and have to be taken while fasting. These drugs have been shown to halt the bone loss caused by long-term use of steroids.

SERMs

For women at risk of osteoporosis who cannot take (or would prefer not to take) HRT, a new category of therapy, selective (o)estrogen receptor modulators (SERMs), may be a solution. Raloxifene is the first SERM to be licensed for use for osteoporosis and it acts in a similar way to tamoxifen, the SERM prescribed for some women to reduce the risk of developing breast cancer. However, it is normally taken by post-menopausal women. Early data suggests that Raloxifene reduces breast cancer, but data about the effects on heart and brain are still awaited as this SERM carries the same DVT (deep vein thrombosis) risks as HRT.

Calcitriol
This is an active form of vitamin D prescribed as Rocaltrol. It has been shown to prevent bone loss but it can result in very high levels of calcium in the blood and urine, which could cause problems. Signs that the levels are too high include nausea, loss of appetite, headaches and fatigue. Too much calcium in the urine could result in kidney stones. As a result, women on Rocaltrol must have their blood and urine carefully monitored.

Heart disease

Although many more men than women suffer from coronary heart disease (CHD) in the 35 to 44 age group, after that the figures even out, so that by the time women reach their mid fifties the risk of CHD starts to increase. Over the age of 75 there is virtually no difference at all between the sexes.

It has taken some time for an older woman's increased risk of heart disease to be recognized, but the figures reveal that although women still live longer than men, 50 per cent of post-menopausal women in Britain die of heart disease as opposed to 8 per cent from breast cancer.

The hormone oestrogen is widely believed to protect women against heart disease before the menopause, which is why post-menopausal women who take HRT seem to be at lower risk. If you have an early menopause, whether natural or surgically induced, you could be at increased risk of CHD if you do not take HRT.

However, your lifestyle also plays an important role. Smoking, too much alcohol, obesity and not exercising all increase your risk of developing heart disease. There is advice about dealing with these issues in Chapter 5. But it's worth bearing in mind, for instance, that even if you are a light smoker you have a higher risk of developing heart disease than a non-smoker, whereas giving up smoking definitely reduces your risk.

Other factors also come into play. If you are diabetic or have high blood pressure these are both implicated in heart disease. Diabetes, which occurs when your body cannot make enough insulin or if the insulin produced is not sufficient to control blood glucose levels, is a major risk factor. The majority of people with diabetes in Britain have Type 2 diabetes (also known as non-insulin dependent diabetes, or NIDD). This develops later in life, which is why it is sometimes also called late-onset diabetes. Although the exact causes still need to be established, a family history of the disease, being of Asian origin, being overweight and doing little exercise all increase your risk.

If you learn to control your diabetes well by keeping to a low fat diet, losing weight, taking exercise and not smoking, you will certainly reduce the chances of CHD. As far as your heart is concerned, one of the problems with diabetes is that it can lead to hardening of the arteries, the large blood vessels that ensure a good supply to the major organs including the heart and kidneys. The risk is greater if you have high blood pressure.

High blood pressure (hypertension) can also develop as you reach middle age. Although there may be no specific cause, there are factors that contribute. Being overweight, taking little or no exercise and too much salt or alcohol in the diet are the main ones. High blood pressure needs to be controlled or treated, because if it is ignored the increased pressure of oxygen-carrying blood going through the arteries can damage them, making them narrow and less flexible. Narrowed arteries mean that organs such as the heart may not receive enough oxygen and, more importantly, it is more likely that a blood clot may form, starving part of the heart or brain of vital oxygen. The result is a heart attack or stroke.

High cholesterol, caused by too much saturated animal fat in the diet, is also believed to play a part in heart disease, as it leads to furring up and narrowing of the arteries. The first-line treatment involves reducing the amount of fats in the diet and increasing exercise and this can be of all-round benefit to the heart.

What you can do

If you know that you have greater chance than most people of developing CHD – for instance, you have a family history of heart disease or have experienced a premature menopause – then you can make sure that you receive the regular checks needed and that, along with everyone else, you make the necessary changes to your lifestyle which have been shown to lower the risk of CHD.

There is an increasing move among some doctors to prescribe HRT to women at particularly high risk of heart disease so if you smoke, have high blood pressure and cholesterol or are diabetic, this is one option that will be suggested and which you might like to consider carefully.

It is also important to see your doctor for regular (annual) blood pressure checks. If your blood pressure is high you may well be tested more often, and if lifestyle changes do not bring it down you may be prescribed beta blockers to keep it under control.

Similarly, if changes in diet do not reduce your cholesterol levels, there are now drugs called statins which can make sure that the levels stay down. Incidentally, there is some early evidence that statins may help to reduce osteoporosis.

Angina

If the coronary arteries are partially blocked this can cause angina – a pain in the chest which can also spread down the arms. It usually occurs after exercise or exertion and subsides after a few minutes of rest, and is caused by insufficient oxygen reaching the heart muscle due to the narrowed arteries. Treatment may be with drugs such as nitrates, which act quickly to dilate the arteries and get the blood flowing through. Beta blockers, also used for high blood pressure, slow the heartbeat as well as reducing blood pressure and allow you to do more before angina starts. Calcium channel blockers also dilate the coronary arteries as well as reducing the rate at which calcium enters the muscles, particularly the heart muscle. You will probably be advised to take a tiny amount of aspirin each day to reduce the risk of a clot forming.

If drugs are not dealing satisfactorily with your symptoms, you may be offered an investigative test called an angiogram followed by a minor operation, angioplasty, to stretch the narrowed coronary arteries. If one or more arteries is blocked then increasingly coronary bypass surgery (CABG) will be performed to replace the blocked arteries.

Helping yourself

There is a great deal that you can do to ensure your heart and arteries remain as healthy as possible.

- Stop smoking.
- Keep your weight under control.
- Take regular exercise.
- Have your blood pressure checked regularly.
- If you are diabetic, keep your blood sugar levels at the right range.
- Eat far less fat of all kinds, but particularly saturated (animal) fats.

For more advice see Chapter 5.

Cancers

As we age we increase our risk of developing cancer. Breast cancer in particular occurs mainly in women over the age of 40, while women over 50 are at higher risk of developing ovarian or uterine cancer. As you get older, there is also an increased chance of cancer of the bowels.

The most important factor with all cancers, apart from prevention, is early diagnosis. Many cancers are either completely curable or at least respond very well to treatment, so it is important to know your body, notice any changes and get them checked without delay.

This is the European Code Against Cancer checklist for possible signs of cancer. See your doctor if you notice any of the following:

- *A lump anywhere in your body* Make a habit of checking your breasts regularly so that you know what they feel like normally. Don't forget to get to know their shape, what your nipples look like, how your breasts change according to the time of the month. From the age of 50 you will be called for breast screening, and this will be repeated every three years. Mammography has already made a huge impact in decreasing mortality from breast cancer in this country. But it also helps to be vigilant because, according to the Cancer Research Campaign, most breast cancers are first spotted either by the person with cancer or by her partner.

- *A change in bowel habits* Again, you need to be familiar with what is normal for you – how often you have a bowel motion, whether your stools are firm or soft. If there are any changes – constipation or diarrhoea, if your stools are black or have blood in them – see your GP just to reassure yourself. Screening for bowel cancer is being tried in some areas to see how effective it may be.

- *Abnormal bleeding* If you bleed between periods it is a sign that something is not quite right. At menopause your periods are likely to be irregular, but any bleeding at other times should be reported to your doctor and investigated. There can be a number of causes for vaginal bleeding – cancer of the womb or cervix may not necessarily be at the top of the list – but you should see your doctor for a diagnosis. If you have not had a period for a year and then experience bleeding you should go to your GP for a full investigation.

You should also see your doctor:

- if you experience unexplained weight loss when you have not been dieting – roughly 5kg or 10lb over a couple of months but this also depends on your normal height and weight;

- if there are any changes in a mole on your skin – such as bleeding, itching, changing shape, size or colour;
- if you have a cough or hoarseness that won't go away.

There are two important changes you can make to your lifestyle to help prevent cancer – stop smoking and eat more healthily. Diet has been linked to several types of cancer, including cancer of the bowel and breast.

You should also attend regular screenings for breast and cervical cancer when you are notified of them. The whole point of screening is to detect a cancer in its early stages when it can be treated much more successfully. There is no organized screening for other cancers, so you need to be vigilant and report any changes that you notice to your doctor.

Fibroids

Fibroids are quite common as women approach the menopause. These growths on or in the wall of the uterus are benign, and if they are small they will be unnoticeable except during a routine pelvic examination. However, if they grow they can cause longer-lasting, painful, heavy periods. A very large fibroid may put pressure on the bladder or bowel. You may feel the lumps in your abdomen and they will certainly show up on an ultrasound scan.

Small fibroids tend to be watched in case they grow but otherwise they are rarely treated. Larger fibroids might need to be removed. Until recently this has involved a hysterectomy, but alternative treatments are being developed that allow them to be treated less invasively using either keyhole surgery or lasers. All fibroids shrivel up at the menopause, unless HRT is given.

Hysterectomy

In the UK each year over 100,000 women (1 in 5) have a hysterectomy, involving the removal of the entire uterus. Most are in their fifties.

In some cases a hysterectomy is a life-saving procedure, used, for instance, to treat cancer in the uterus, ovaries, Fallopian tubes or cervix or an advanced infection in the pelvis. In other circumstances, for example to treat large fibroids or very heavy periods, there is an increasing feeling that many of these operations are unnecessary.

Alternatives such as the Mirena coil or endometrial ablation (using laser, a heated wire loop or a microwave technique to remove the womb lining) are also available. If a specialist suggests a hysterectomy, you should always discuss the matter carefully both with him and with your own GP, as well as informing yourself as much as possible, before agreeing.

Many surgeons will still routinely remove the ovaries while performing a hysterectomy, on the basis that in an older woman 'they are no longer needed' and their removal lowers the risk of ovarian cancer. But unless the ovaries are diseased or there is a family history of ovarian cancer, there is no logical reason to perform this procedure and it becomes a matter of personal choice. You will continue to ovulate but you will not have periods. Your menopause may start earlier. If your ovaries are removed you will experience symptoms of the menopause, and most women in this situation are offered HRT.

Make sure you discuss your wishes with the gynaecologist before surgery and ask why your ovaries need to be removed. Ask about possible after-effects, such as loss of libido, premature ovarian failure (30 per cent of ovaries kept following a hysterectomy fail within two years) and whether there are any other non-surgical options. If necessary seek a second opinion before signing any consent form.

Urinary problems

It is quite common to have urinary problems at the menopause – especially post-menopause. It is equally common to keep this to yourself, feeling far too embarrassed to mention it to anyone else, even those closest to you.

Incontinence

We have already looked at incontinence in Chapter 2, but it is such a common problem that it is worth discussing again here.

Weakness of the muscle at the neck of the bladder which controls the flow of urine is the cause of many of the problems. These include urgency – when the urge to pass urine is so sudden that you may not get to the toilet in time – and frequency, which is when you constantly feel the need to go to the toilet.

Stress incontinence is something that can affect women of all ages – it is reckoned that around 80 per cent of women will suffer from it at some stage in their lives, but it is much more common at this time.

You may find that you leak urine or even experience an embarrassing flood when you laugh, cough, try to lift something or exercise. It is the result of weak muscles in the pelvic floor, triggered by childbirth, by strenuous exercise such as weight-lifting and by some of the changes that take place in the body at the menopause.

The problem is that many women suffer incontinence of this kind in silence (and you could well be among them) because they are too embarrassed to talk to their doctor or may assume that there is nothing that can be done. Without any treatment, incontinence can really affect your quality of life. You may find it difficult to arrange outings, and even going shopping can become a major excursion. You may feel uncomfortable in front of other people in case there is a smell; you may spend your days changing your underwear, and your sex life can also be affected if you wet the bed at night.

There are some good products on the market that will give you the protection you need. They are similar to sanitary towels but offer much better absorption of larger amounts of liquid so there is no risk of an 'accident'.

However, if you can overcome your embarrassment and go for advice, you will find that there is plenty of help and support available, including pelvic floor exercises to strengthen the pelvic muscle (see Chapter 2 for instructions), which can improve or cure most stress incontinence.

There are also vaginal weights, small cones to place in the vagina, rather like tampons. You start with a lightweight cone to hold in place; as the muscles get stronger, you can insert slightly heavier cones. You may find these helpful if you are not sure you are doing your pelvic floor exercises correctly.

Inferential therapy uses electrical impulses to exercise the muscle. Collagen injections (known as Contigen) may be used to build up tissue around the bladder. Other therapies include medicines which can control urinary flow and a PVC ring which can be used by older women after the menopause to stabilize and support the urethra. In some cases, surgery may be suggested to strengthen weak muscles.

If you really don't want to talk to your doctor, there are helplines you can contact anonymously for advice and help (see Useful Addresses).

Urinary infections and thrush

It is believed that the fall in oestrogen levels makes women more vulnerable to infections such as cystitis. The symptoms include a burning sensation when you pass urine, needing to go to the toilet more often, pain in the lower abdomen and urine that smells. If you have never had cystitis before, it's important to see your doctor for a proper diagnosis as soon as possible. If the symptoms are treated in the early stages there is a better chance that you will suffer only the one bout.

The doctor will need to take a sample of urine, not only to diagnose the cystitis but also to establish which particular bacterium has caused the infection. She will then be able to prescribe a course of the appropriate antibiotics.

Both during the infection and later, after the cystitis has cleared up, there are some simple things you can do to help yourself:

- avoid using any soap products around the genital area;
- drink as much water as you can each day – around four pints is ideal – to dilute any bacteria that may be present in the bladder;
- get into the habit, when you wipe yourself after going to the toilet, of wiping from front to back rather than the other way round, to reduce the risk of infection passing from the rectal area;
- cranberry juice, also available as tablets, has helped many women keep their cystitis attacks at bay. It has been shown to have a specific chemical in it that stops E. coli, the bacterium that causes cystitis, from holding on to the inside lining of your bladder. Drink 30ml last thing at night.

Thrush is a yeast infection and is also common at this time – three out of four women will get thrush at some stage in their lives. The symptoms are swelling of the vaginal area accompanied by intense itchiness. There is also a vaginal discharge which is thick, white and a bit like curds. Thrush is not a sexually transmitted disease; it arises when the balance of the bacteria and yeasts that live naturally in the vagina is disturbed and one type of yeast, candida albicans, breeds faster than usual, making the area too alkaline. Antibiotics, oral contraceptives, hormonal changes that take place during menstruation, pregnancy and at the menopause, diabetes and stress are all known to play a part.

It is important to see your GP to get the thrush properly diagnosed if this is your first bout, but treatments can either be prescribed or bought over the counter. There are pills such as Diflucan which can clear thrush in a matter of days. You can also buy pessaries and creams. Remember that men can get thrush, too, and that it's easily passed on during intercourse, so if your thrush keeps recurring your partner or spouse should also be treated.

You can help yourself by following the advice for cystitis (above).

The following tips are also useful when dealing with thrush.

- Wear cotton underwear and avoid tight-fitting tights or trousers as thrush thrives in a moist, warm environment.
- Plain, live yoghurt applied outside and inside the vagina works well for many women to reduce the itching and soreness, as does pure aloe vera juice.
- Herbal creams such as calendula may help to reduce the itching.

Keeping your health in check

Most GP surgeries now have 'Well Woman' clinics. Depending on the system you may either be called in for a check or make your own appointment.

The clinic is run by either the practice nurse or the family doctor. They will check your blood pressure and carry out a cervical smear test, if required. You will have been asked to bring along a urine sample which will be screened for diabetes; blood may be taken to look at your cholesterol levels, to see if you are anaemic and to check thyroid function. You will be measured and weighed and your body mass index will be calculated.

This is the ideal time to ask questions and get advice. The nurse can help if you want to lose weight, give up smoking or take more exercise. If you are concerned about your calcium intake or whether you need additional vitamins or supplements, she will be able to advise on your diet. You can discuss areas such as breast screening or a bone-density scan. The nurse will also ask you questions about your lifestyle to find out what extra pressures there are in your life. Maybe you have elderly parents to look after, have young children or even grandchildren to care for, or a full- or part-time job.

You may also feel more comfortable asking her questions about some of your other symptoms such as incontinence, thrush or vaginal dryness. If you have symptoms that worry you, such as bleeding between periods or after intercourse or unexplained lumps in your breasts, these can be investigated further – first by your family doctor and then, if necessary, by a specialist.

Essential tests

Breast screening
Screening is an important way in which possible problems can be detected in the early stages, when successful treatment is much more likely. From the age of 50 you will be offered breast screening and recalled every three years. Usually this will be held at a local

hospital, a special unit or in a mobile breast-screening unit. A mammography (breast X-ray) takes very little time. On arrival your name and details will be checked; you will then be asked to take off all the clothes on your top half, including your bra – usually a dressing gown is provided or you may put on your jacket or coat. During the mammography each breast in turn is spread and gently pressed in order to see it in detail. Some women do find this quite uncomfortable, but it lasts for only a few seconds. If your breasts are very tender then try and make sure your next appointment doesn't coincide with that time of the month. The results take up to two weeks to come through. Around 5 women in 100 have to return, either for more tests – in which case you will be told the results at once – or for another X-ray if the one taken is not clear enough to be read.

A mammography can't pick up everything, so being breast aware is still important. Examine your breasts regularly so that you get to know how they usually look and feel.

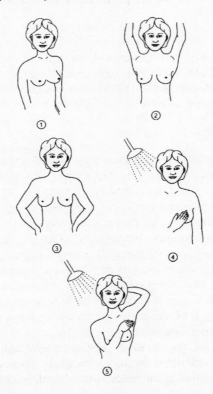

Be breast aware

Check your breasts once every month or two. The ideal time is in the week after a period, or at the same time of each month if your periods have finished.

- Stand in front of the mirror and examine both your breasts from all angles. Look at the nipples – have they changed at all? Are they darker? (1)
- With both arms above your head, look and see if there are any differences. (2)
- With hands on hips pushing inwards, look at the breasts again, both from the sides and underneath. (3) Now, lean forward and get to know the shape of your breasts so you can notice any changes.
- Feel for any changes within the breast – this is easier done in the shower or bath with a soapy hand. Work your way round each breast, pressing lightly as you go. (4)
- Feel along towards the armpit to see if there is anything different in that area. (5)

Cervical smear

Have regular tests, as these will reveal any early signs of abnormality. Early treatment of cervical cancer is completely successful, so if you are or have been sexually active this is an important screening to have.

And not forgetting . . .

- The most common eye problem for women from the age of 40 onwards is presbyopia – far-sightedness. As you get older the shape of the eye's lens gradually changes and it gets harder to focus. Have an annual eye check from now on to make sure you have the prescription glasses that you need. There is also a test for glaucoma – a condition that occurs when the drainage of fluid from inside the eye is impaired. It is treatable once diagnosed, but left untreated it can cause loss of vision and eventually blindness.
- Your hearing should remain good for many years to come, but you may find it a little harder to hear higher-pitched sounds. If you are finding it harder to hear – mumbling teenagers excluded – then talk to your doctor.
- Taking care of the teeth is just as important now. At the menopause women are far more likely to develop gum disease (pyorrhoea). If this is untreated, teeth become loose and have to

be removed. See the dentist twice a year for a check-up and the dental hygienist at least three times a year to have your teeth thoroughly cleaned. In between, use a toothbrush properly to brush in a circular motion where teeth and gums meet, and use dental floss twice a day to clean between teeth.

- You are still going to expect your feet to carry you, so take care of them. Keep toe nails short, cutting straight across and not down the sides. See a chiropodist for any corns or bunions, and if you are diabetic see the doctor if you notice any cuts or breaks in the skin. If you plan to do more walking or exercise, make sure you have the right shoes to reduce the risk of blisters.

5

Looking after yourself

This is the time in your life when you need to put yourself first. Paying some attention to your overall physical and emotional health is worth it. It will not only help you cope better with the menopause but, just as important, it will give you the resources to remain healthy in the years to come.

Nothing can stop us getting older chronologically, but there is a lot we can do to justify the saying that 'You're only as old as you feel.' It is possible to slow down some of the ageing processes and delay the development of many conditions, such as osteoarthritis, heart disease and breathing problems, that are in some cases life-threatening and at the very least can make the post-menopausal years difficult by limiting what you can do and preventing you from living life to the full.

Changing habits

There are some habits that, as you get older, put you at a much higher risk of long-term illness or premature death, namely smoking, drinking and over-eating. Now is the time to break those bad habits, if you possibly can.

Smoking

In women cases of lung cancer are rising, while in men the rate is falling. Lung cancer is now a bigger killer of women than breast cancer in the UK. Whichever way you look at it, smoking is a pretty destructive habit. There are links with a whole range of cancers – lung, throat and mouth, cervical, bladder and kidney are the most common. Smokers are twice as likely to experience respiratory problems, such as wheezing, breathlessness and coughing, compared to non-smokers. The longer you have been smoking, the more likely you are to have these symptoms, and even if your daily tally of cigarettes is the same as a man's, you are more likely to have breathing problems. Although no one is absolutely sure why, it is believed that women are more vulnerable because they have smaller airways, exposing them to higher levels of the poisonous substances in cigarettes than men. There are also the increased risks of developing heart problems, circulatory diseases such as chronic bronchitis and emphysema, and cancers of the mouth, throat and lungs.

Female smokers have lower bone density than non-smokers because they often have a lower intake of vitamin D and calcium – both essential for healthy bones and bone formation – and so are at higher risk of developing osteoporosis. Women smokers also tend to have an earlier menopause (by two years on average) and some symptoms, such as hot flushes, are much stronger. After the menopause, if you are not on HRT, as a smoker you are at greater risk of a heart attack or stroke and, on a purely aesthetic level, your skin is far more likely to be wrinkled, especially around the mouth, and your teeth and fingers are likely to be discoloured.

Giving up

No one would claim that it's easy to give up smoking, even if you know all the risks. You have probably tried several times already. However, you are far more likely to be successful and stay a non-smoker if you make the decision to stop entirely on your own, rather than responding to your family nagging you or even your doctor advising you to stop.

The way you stop smoking is very personal – what works for one person may not work for another. It will help if you remember that the positive benefits of stopping smoking start very soon after you stub out that final cigarette.

This is what happens when you stop smoking:

- in 20 minutes blood pressure and pulse rate return to normal;
- in 8 hours nicotine and carbon monoxide levels in the blood are reduced by half, and oxygen levels return to normal;
- in 24 hours carbon monoxide is eliminated from the body, and lungs start to clear out mucus and other smoking debris;
- in 48 hours there is no nicotine left in your body; you can taste and smell much better;
- in 72 hours your breathing becomes easier;
- in 3–9 months your lung function will have increased by up to 10 per cent;
- in 5 years your risk of heart attack falls to half that of a smoker;
- in 10 years your risk of lung cancer is half that of a smoker and your risk of a heart attack is the same as someone who has never smoked.

© Health Authority/NUS

Good ways to quit

When you really think about it, you may find that your smoking is no longer for enjoyment and that you are using it as a crutch – maybe to reduce stress or to help you concentrate. You might not even be conscious of lighting up – it's such an automatic response. Some ex-smokers have found it easier to go 'cold turkey' and stop from one day to the next, while others need more time. Cutting down to around five cigarettes a day may be an option – but it rarely works in the long term. Various 'aids' can help: nicotine patches or gum (but, remember, you will still be getting a small nicotine fix and this may become another habit to break); hypnotherapy; acupuncture; group therapy. There is also a new drug, Zyban, which seems effective, but it is only available on prescription from your surgery and there is some concern about risks involved in taking it. These and other therapies can be very successful, not just at getting you to stop but also, even more important, at keeping you stopped.

Allen Carr, who runs highly successful 'stop smoking' clinics, believes that the answer lies in telling yourself that you are not an ex-smoker but a non-smoker, and that once you make that decision to smoke your last cigarette you are free from a very addictive habit. The government-funded agency Quit has a helpline and a useful website (see Useful Addresses, p. 111). In the end, though, you must choose the method that works best for you – and don't be discouraged if at first you fail. Each time you make the attempt to quit, you are one step nearer to finally being a non-smoker.

I'd given up smoking several times but I'd always started again. One day I read an article in a newspaper about someone who'd stopped smoking using acupuncture. I was inspired to try by the fact that the writer claimed that she felt wonderful for the first three days. I found a local acupuncturist and made an appointment for first thing in the morning. She spent quite some time talking to me about my smoking habits – why I smoked, when I smoked most and so on. Then I simply lay down and she placed needles in my ankles – to relax me, she explained – and a stud at the top of each ear. If I felt the need to smoke I had to press the studs. I left feeling really relaxed, and I felt on top of the world for three days. Then the cravings hit me but I pressed the studs and sucked barley sugars like mad for the next two weeks. After a fortnight the studs were taken out. By then the cravings were less, but I returned for two further sessions when she simply gave me a relaxing massage. That was 12 years ago and I haven't wanted or smoked a cigarette since.

Alcohol

Having the occasional drink is absolutely fine – a glass of wine in the evening, even two, will relax you after a long day. It's sociable, too. Initially, alcohol makes you feel relaxed and happy. However, too much alcohol can increase the risk of many physical problems.

Alcohol affects the brain – even moderate drinking can cause the loss of some brain cells. Heavy drinking can damage the liver so that it can no longer process the nutrients in food nor eliminate toxins from the blood; women are at higher risk of this and can develop liver disease at lower levels of drinking. Alcohol is one of the main causes of high blood pressure and increases the risk of some cancers, notably of the gullet and the liver. It can cause digestive problems such as gastritis and stomach bleeding.

However, although heavy drinking may affect your organs, the main risk is to the brain. Scans of the brains of women who drink heavily – and women generally are drinking far more alcohol than they used to – show that brain tissue has shrunk. In tests these women performed less well in terms of memory, speed of response, reasoning and perception. Heavy drinking can also lead to vitamin deficiency and liver disease.

Around the time of the menopause some women may begin to drink more heavily. It may be as an escape, as a way to relieve stress, depression or boredom, but it doesn't work. In fact, alcohol in excess heightens those feelings, especially depression. Far from helping you to sleep, alcohol actually causes insomnia and can make things worse if you already have difficulty sleeping. It's often hard to recognize, let alone admit to yourself that you are drinking too much. Most heavy drinkers are very good at hiding the amount they consume. However, once you do recognize the problem you are in a strong position to do something about it.

The current recommended alcohol consumption for women (who absorb alcohol differently from men) is no more than two to three units a day, and no more than 14 units a week. A unit is equivalent to a glass of wine (125ml), one measure of spirits (25ml) or a half-pint of beer (250ml). A heavy drinker will regularly consume ten units a day. You need to bear in mind that, if you drink at home, unless you use a measure you are likely to pour yourself more than a unit.

Research has shown that regular drinkers (i.e. those who drink every night of the week) are at higher risk of damaging their liver that those who have their units more irregularly. As a woman, if you regularly drink three units a night you will increasingly be putting your health at risk.

To discover whether you need to be concerned about how much alcohol you are drinking, ask yourself the following questions:

Do you:

- get drunk more often these days?
- have to take time off work because of a hangover?
- have accidents, arguments or injuries because of drink?
- invariably drink more than you planned in an evening?
- think a lot about when you can next have a drink?

If you are experiencing any of the above or are not sure what your alcohol intake might be, then it is a good idea to try to keep a diary for a fairly typical week, noting down the amount you drink and when. It will give you a clear idea of what is going on, and you will be able to take steps to cut down if you can see that you are drinking above the recommended limits.

On the other hand, if you already know you are drinking more than is safe, see if any of the following statements apply to you:

- If I don't have a drink every day, I do miss it.
- I always gulp down my first drink.
- I am always the first person to finish a drink.
- I often have a hangover.
- I need a drink before certain events or situations.
- In the morning or middle of the night I have the shakes or sweat.
- I spend more than I can afford on alcohol.
- I order doubles when it's my round.
- I often feel that I need a drink.
- I get annoyed if others mention my drinking.
- I feel secretly uncomfortable about my drinking.
- I drink earlier in the day.

According to Alcohol Concern, you are likely to have a definite problem with alcohol or have become addicted if you:

- have to increase the amount you drink to maintain the same effect;
- always wake up with the shakes and feeling sweaty;
- need a drink to start the day;
- drink large quantities over the course of the day without it making you drunk;
- feel uncomfortable if you don't have a drink at hand;

- lie about your drinking;
- are covering up your drinking and the costs of it.

What you can do

- Try to have that first drink later.
- Replace alcoholic drinks with soft drinks or low-alcohol drinks.
- Don't have quick drinks during your lunch-hour or after work.
- Organize yourself so that you have at least two alcohol-free days each week – taking up a sport or some other new interest can help.
- Choose longer drinks – you may drink less if you have cider or beer rather than spirits – and drink them more slowly.
- If you drink at home, buy smaller glasses or a drinks measure so that you can watch the number of units.
- Tell friends and family that you are cutting down.
- Find other ways of relaxing – for example, exercise or relaxation techniques.

Going for help

Check in your local telephone book under Alcohol.

Drinkline can offer you help and advice and details of your local service. Call 0800 917 82 82 (freephone).

Alcohol Concern publishes leaflets and booklets. *A Woman's Guide to Alcohol* will answer many of your questions. Single copies are free from Alcohol Concern (see Useful Addresses, p. 109).

Weight control

Obesity is a growing problem in Britain today, with 53 per cent of women (and 62 per cent of men) classified as overweight, and 17 per cent of women (20 per cent of men) as obese. This is usually calculated using the body mass index (see p. 67).

Being overweight may mean you have a later menopause (and fewer wrinkles on your face), but against this you are at higher risk of heart disease, high blood pressure, hip and knee problems (as they struggle to support the extra weight), diabetes and certain cancers.

Most women do experience some weight gain around the menopause, but it is not inevitable. Your metabolic rate slows from your forties onwards, so you need fewer calories to function. This means that if you carry on eating as much as you always have (or more) and do not take any regular exercise, your body won't use up the extra calories and you'll put on weight. More importantly, it is known that, as oestrogen levels fall, the way fat is stored round the body changes from being around the hips and thighs to being stored round the abdomen. This means that an overweight woman's shape at the menopause becomes more like that of a man. Research shows that men with large stomachs are at higher risk of heart attack, and the same applies to women.

If you have always had a weight problem, the solution may be more complex than simply eating less, as evidence suggests that there is more to it than just eating too much. For many people, that extra weight can be due to their metabolic rate (the energy your body uses to perform functions like breathing, digesting food, keeping a regular heartbeat), family traditions and even heredity. Some women blame HRT for their weight gain, but there is little evidence that this is the case – in fact the opposite may occur, because with increased oestrogens body fat will tend to stay around the hips and thighs rather than the waist.

You'll probably be more than aware of whether you are overweight or not, but a useful guide is to calculate your body mass index (BMI) which shows the ratio of fat you are carrying around. First work out your height in metres and your weight in kilograms. Then divide your weight by your height squared. For instance, say you are 1.6 metres tall and weight 65kg. The sum looks like this: $1.6 \times 1.6 = 2.56$. Then 65 divided by $2.56 = 25.39$. If your BMI is between 20 and 25, then your weight is right for your height. If your BMI is between 25 and 30 then you are overweight. A BMI of over 30 means that you are obese. You may find the current advice for women, whatever their height, easier to follow. If your waistline measures more than 80cm (32in) you should try to lose a few pounds. If your waistline is bigger than 88cm (35in) you should see your doctor and discuss ways in which your excess weight can be lost.

What you can do
Even if you lose just a little weight you can reduce high blood pressure and lower your cholesterol level, so if you decide to lose some weight at this stage in your life you will not only improve your overall health but will also look better and feel more confident and in control. If your weight gain is considerable, you should see your doctor for advice. It also helps to lose weight with others, so think about joining a local club or getting together with friends. It often helps to have someone with whom you can share your successes and failures, exchange ideas and encourage each other to keep going.

I'd had a real problem with my weight ever since the birth of my second child. I was always trying one diet or another. As I hit my mid-forties my weight really increased and I started to feel so fed up with myself. I saw a small ad in the post office for a group that was starting in the village hall. We weren't following any particular scheme. We used a sort of 'eat less, weigh less' diet from a women's magazine, and we all paid something towards the hire of the hall. It was just a group of local women who wanted to lose weight. We set our own targets and encouraged each other. Some of us met up in between to exercise or walk. It was a slow process and there were times when I felt really discouraged, but the advantage of a village group is that you keep meeting up at other times, so it's a lot harder to opt out. We all lost weight, and although I've had the odd hiccup I've never gained more than a few pounds, and it's been easier to lose it again.

Losing weight safely

The most effective way to lose weight is to eat fewer calories. If at the same time you exercise regularly, you should lose around 500g/1lb a week. For some women reducing calories may mean skipping meals, using meal replacements and other over-the-counter products as well as calorie counting. Crash diets, drastically reducing your calorie intake over a short period, don't work. You will lose weight but the evidence is that you will regain as much as two-thirds of the weight lost within a year. Ninety per cent of those who go on crash diets regain the weight they have lost, plus a bit more, within a couple of years.

There are also risks associated with very low-calorie diets of less than 1,000 calories a day. As well as risking a vitamin and mineral deficiency, you may lose lean body mass as well as fat. You increase your chances of bone loss by upsetting your hormonal balance. Drugs such as Xenecal (orlistat) are now coming on to the market, which can absorb as much as 30 per cent of the fat you eat – but so far they are only available on prescription and can only be used under supervision. They may be a solution for patients with a BMI of over 30, who cannot lose weight by eating less and exercising.

Getting into exercise

Exercise on its own may not help you to lose weight, but alongside a reduced-calorie diet it can help you to lose a little extra and if you continue to exercise, the weight is more likely to stay off (see more about exercise below). You will also find that you can achieve a trimmer, more toned figure. Research shows that people who include physical activity in their weight-loss programmes are more likely to keep their weight off than people who only change their diet and they also improve their bone density.

Several studies have shown that to lose weight successfully you need to set realistic, even modest goals and take it slowly – this increases your chances of losing weight and not regaining it. The best and safest method is to make a long-term change in your lifestyle, in what you eat and how much.

Eating well

Food provides us with the essential nutrients our bodies need to function well, and this is especially important during the menopause, when there is every opportunity to lay a good foundation for the years to come. The key word is balance: not eating too much or too little of anything, but making sure that you include a wide variety of essential nutrients – proteins, carbohydrates, fats, vitamins, minerals and trace elements.

A balanced diet is essential for cell renewal, for a healthy immune system to protect us against illness and disease, for joints and muscles to continue to function well. But at the time of the menopause it's especially important to focus on the areas most at risk now – heart and bones. A few minor changes can make a real difference.

Look after your heart

At menopause women gradually lose the extra protection provided by oestrogen, and their risk of heart disease becomes similar to that for men (see Chapter 4). You can protect your heart by stopping smoking, cutting down on alcohol, taking regular exercise (see below) and by eating a little more carefully. In particular, reduce the amount of fat, salt and sugar in your diet.

Build strong bones

Both women and men begin to lose bone mass from their mid-thirties onwards, but at menopause this loss increases because the body lacks the hormone oestrogen which helps to maintain bone strength by drawing calcium into the bones. There is no cure for osteoporosis, so prevention is important. As well as exercise, your bones need a good supply of calcium – around 1200mg a day, ideally from natural sources such as milk, yoghurt, oily fish, dried apricots and broccoli.

If you are sure you are not getting enough calcium then take a supplement – choose one that includes vitamin D and magnesium as they both help the calcium to be absorbed better.

Care for your digestion

Many women experience constipation during the menopause, so a good amount of roughage in your diet – from wholegrain cereals, pulses, dark green leafy vegetables, nuts and seeds – can be helpful. These foods also make you feel more satisfied, which in turn makes it easier to control your appetite. You should also drink plenty of water – an average of around two litres a day. Some of it will come from fruit and vegetables, but the rest should either be pure water, unsweetened fruit juices or low-fat milk. Drinks like tea, coffee or colas, that seem to contain a lot of water, also contain caffeine, which acts as a diuretic, increasing the amount of water lost. Cola drinks are also high in phosphates, which displace calcium, so they are not helpful to bones.

Hormonal changes or HRT can trigger intolerance to foods that you may have eaten quite happily until now. If you are experiencing symptoms such as diarrhoea, sickness, gut pain, bloating, migraine, extreme fatigue or constipation, your digestive system may be trying to tell you something.

There is no doubt that we are becoming increasingly sensitive to some foods – especially those that contain additives or have been sprayed with pesticides or other chemicals. Antibiotics given to animals and poultry can also be passed into the human digestive system and upset the balance of flora in the gut.

These reactions to certain foods are often hard to diagnose, and if you are already experiencing irritability and fatigue as a symptom of the menopause, you might not even think of the food you eat as a possible additional cause. However, it is worth considering, especially if you do suffer a lot of bloating and other bowel-related problems. The most common foods that seem to cause intolerance these days among adults are dairy products and wheat. At this age it can simply be that your body has reached its limit in terms of a certain food. In the case of wheat, in particular, if you have cereal and toast for breakfast, a sandwich for lunch and pasta in the evening, you will have eaten a lot of wheat.

Naturally you will want to check any symptoms with your doctor, but if you feel that certain foods may be making you feel unwell or uncomfortable, you can try keeping a food diary over two or three weeks, writing down what you eat and how you feel. This way you may be able to pinpoint the culprit(s). Once you have done this you can try removing a specific food from your diet and see how you feel over a week or two. In the case of wheat, you can replace it with other cereals such as rye or millet, and you can substitute soya, goat or sheep's milk for cow's milk. If there are no major digestive problems you may find that simply eating as much fresh food as possible can help you to feel a lot more comfortable.

Prevent cancer

A high-fibre diet which includes plenty of fresh fruit and vegetables is believed to reduce the risk of some cancers – especially of the breast and colon. You also need to have a good supply of the antioxidant vitamins E and C. If you follow the advice on caring for your digestive system, you can also protect your body against these cancers.

Know the guidelines

Although there has been some confusion in the past, the healthy eating guidelines for a balanced diet have been streamlined and are now much easier to understand and make part of your life.

- Have at least five portions of vegetables and/or fruit a day, fresh or frozen, preferably raw or steamed. Eat plenty of dark green vegetables such as broccoli, spinach or cabbage. Snack on carrot or celery sticks, bananas, apples and other fresh fruit.
- Eat a good amount of starchy foods such as bread, rice, pasta, (preferably wholegrain) and potatoes. These contain natural sugars which are released slowly to give sustained energy.
- Include some dairy products such as skimmed milk, yoghurt and cottage cheese to ensure you have enough calcium (1200mg a day) in your diet. If you cannot tolerate dairy products then you can get the amount of calcium you need from a good supplement.
- Eat far less saturated fat from meat products. If you eat meat, trim off visible fat. Use olive oil instead of butter. Try to have a meat meal no more than twice a week.
- Eat fish – at least three times a week. Oily fish – salmon, mackerel, herring, sardines – contain Omega-3 fatty acids which can help reduce the risk of heart disease. Other fish are a good source of protein and are low in fat, provided you do not fry them or cover them in a cream sauce.
- Get some protein from non-animal sources – beans, lentils and other pulses such as soya.
- Cut down on salt to control your blood pressure. As well as eating

fewer salty foods, add as little salt as possible to your meals and don't put salt on the table. Herbs and spices can be used instead to add flavour.

- Cut down on sugar to protect your teeth, keep your weight stable and reduce the risk of developing Type II diabetes.
- Grill, steam or bake food rather than frying or boiling. There is less fat and you retain more nutrients.

Keeping active

Exercise is important at all stages of life, but if we want to remain active as we get older it is increasingly a case of 'use it or lose it'. For women at the menopause, regular exercise can make a tremendous difference in both the short and long term.

Exercise can help control the weight increase that can occur at this time, although if you already exercise, and continue to eat the same amount, you may find you need to do more exercise (and eat a bit less!) to maintain the status quo. It can also alleviate menopausal symptoms. Hot flushes and night sweats may not be so ferocious or frequent, and regular movement will reduce muscular aches and pains.

In the long term, regular exercise will reduce your risk of heart disease, stroke, diabetes and osteoporosis, and lower your blood pressure and cholesterol levels. You will lose fat and build up lean body mass such as muscle. You will also find that your overall mood improves, you will feel less stressed and more positive about life and yourself. You will also sleep better and feel less anxious/depressed, and you may find it easier to concentrate and think clearly.

One of the immediate effects of exercise is to release endorphins in the brain. These chemical neurotransmitters give you a special sense of well-being, usually just when you finish an exercise session. They can make you feel on top of the world.

You are probably quite keen to exercise, so here are some tips before you get started:

- Choose an exercise that is right for you. Don't choose an activity because it's popular or trendy. If you don't enjoy it you will find it harder and harder to keep up.
- Start slowly and build up gradually. There is far less risk of injury this way.
- Exercise in a group or with a friend for support and encouragement.
- Do a variety of different exercises – this is called cross-training. It

will prevent you getting bored but will also make sure that every part of your body is being exercised and nothing is being put under too much stress.

- Always warm up the muscles in the arms and legs before and after exercise to reduce the risk of strains and sprains.
- Lead a more active life in general – make exercise as much a part of your life as brushing your teeth every day.
- Have fun – exercise should be something you enjoy!

How to keep going

Starting to exercise is easy, it's keeping the exercise going that is hard. Most people start out full of enthusiasm, but unless you have a set yourself some short- and long-term goals you will find it really hard to maintain your exercise and sustain your initial enthusiasm.

Your goals need to be realistic. For instance, to start with you may set yourself a three-month goal of being able to exercise aerobically for 20 minutes without getting too out of breath. A long-term goal might be to take part in a 3km walk or to swim 30 lengths of the pool for your favourite charity.

It will also help to have a specific time of day for your exercise – obviously there will be some flexibility but you need to work out when you function at your best. For instance, if you have more energy in the morning and the house is quiet, then that's probably the best time for you to exercise. On the other hand, if you are at work you may find early evening works better.

If you miss an exercise session, don't worry too much but try to get back into the routine as soon as you can.

Listen to your body

Stop if you have any pain, feel dizzy or sick or are very short of breath. You should also stop if your heart rate doesn't slow down after five minutes or if your pulse is irregular.

When you are exercising you need to feel that you are working the various areas of your body. You will breathe faster and harder, but if you feel very out of breath then you should slow down and reduce the pace.

In the early stages it is normal to have some muscle soreness after exercise but you shouldn't have any pain. If there is pain then you have probably done too much, too soon. Take things back a stage until you are ready to move on.

Every January I promised myself that this would be the year when I started exercising regularly, but somehow it never quite happened. I joined classes at the local gym but stopped going after a few weeks; I tried to go swimming but never quite got into the rhythm, so that fizzled out as well. I mentioned this to a friend and she felt the same way – she also wanted to exercise regularly but had found it really hard to keep going. We decided to start together and for the first six months we treated ourselves to a personal trainer. She was brilliant because she assessed us beforehand, produced a programme for us to follow each week and gradually increased the level of what we could do safely. We also had to keep a daily diary of what we had done. Knowing that once a week we would see her made it easier to do the exercise, and after six months we were ready to go it alone – it was enough time for exercise to be part of the weekly routine.

Making the most of it

To achieve a good overall level of fitness, you need to exercise in three specific ways to improve your stamina, strength and suppleness. If you haven't exercised for some time, are very overweight or have medical problems, you should always check with your doctor before starting regular exercise.

Stamina

These are the aerobic exercises that work on the cardiovascular system by raising the heart rate and making you breathe faster. It will mean you can keep going for longer without getting exhausted or feeling totally out of breath. As well as benefiting the heart and lungs, aerobic exercise often improves digestion too. Choose any activity that you enjoy, but it must be fairly vigorous – brisk walking, dancing, jogging, an aerobics class, even housework or gardening. Start with 10 to 15 minutes of exercise and build up to 20 or 30 minutes of your chosen activity three to five times a week, at a level that makes you breathe faster but doesn't make you breathless – you should be able to continue to hold a conversation. These activities also have the advantage of being weight-bearing, so they will help to maintain bone mass. Before you start, do a gentle five-minute warm-up with some jogging on the spot and a few stretches of calf, thigh and leg muscles.

Strength

Strong muscles mean that you can carry on performing everyday tasks without injury or strain. Toned muscles will give you a better shape as well as reducing the chances of conditions such as back pain.

The exercises you can do for yourself at home will include strengthening muscles in your stomach, thighs, and arms.

Most local leisure centres now have gyms with weight-training equipment, specifically designed to help you improve your muscle tone. Book in for an assessment with a trained fitness instructor and get a programme worked out for your level of fitness. If you prefer to exercise at home, some press-ups against the wall will help strengthen upper arms while squats work on the thighs and leg muscles.

Suppleness
Working on flexibility now means that in the years to come you will be able to bend, stretch and reach as efficiently as possible. The best exercises for improving suppleness involve stretching various areas of the body – reaching up and out to the side with your arms, gentle twists of the upper body from one side to the other, and so on. Most exercise classes include stretching exercises in a session, but if you really enjoy this type of exercise you may find that yoga is the perfect choice, combining postures that improve both suppleness and strength.

Managing stress

We all need some element of stress in our lives to push us into action, but there is a world of difference between an exciting new challenge that fires you with enthusiasm and a certain amount of trepidation and the sort of stress that prevents you from sleeping at night and gives you headaches, backache, palpitations or medical problems such as irritable bowel syndrome.

Life during the menopause can be stressful for all sorts of reasons. You may have concerns about work, children, relationships, elderly parents. Then there are the symptoms of the menopause to contend with, plus your own thoughts about the present and future. It's hardly surprising that a lot of women at this time just feel like walking out of the front door and running away from it all. There may be very little you can do to change the external sources of your stress and coming to terms with that is an achievement in itself – but what you can do is train yourself to react and deal with these problems in a more relaxed way.

For many women, one of the first things to learn at this stage of life is the art of delegation. If you have spent the past 20-odd years running the whole show, now is the time to stand back a little and stop trying to do everything yourself. As you take that step back from being superwoman and practise saying 'no' occasionally, you might also realize that some things are not absolutely essential anyway – and can be left undone or at least delayed.

Guilt is an emotion that drives many women these days as they try to juggle several lives, but however busy you are, try to make time for yourself each day. It need not be very long – half an hour is ideal, but ten totally uninterrupted minutes are better than nothing. During that time sit quietly, read, listen to some music, have a bath, go for a walk – anything you enjoy that allows you to switch off for a while. Every so often, give yourself a proper treat. Go to the theatre with a friend, have a massage, a facial, a new hairdo. Enjoy life!

Learning to relax

Meditation or deep relaxation can be a very useful way to switch off for a while. It takes time to learn to stop thoughts intruding, but focusing on relaxing the body is a good first step.

A simple relaxation exercise

Wear loose, comfortable clothes, take off shoes and socks/tights. Make sure you are warm enough.

Lie on the floor on a mat or folded blanket. Support your head with a pillow if it feels more comfortable, and place a folded towel under your knees if you feel tense when your legs are straight.

Let your feet roll out and your arms lie a little distance away from your body, palms facing upwards.

Feel your whole body gradually relax and sink into the floor. Some people like to work their way round – feet, legs, thighs, buttocks, back, hands, arms, shoulders, neck, head – tensing and releasing each part to feel the difference. Make sure that your palms are open, fingers relaxed. Feel your shoulders move down away from your head and into the floor. Close your eyes, but don't squeeze them shut, and completely relax your jaw – your teeth should not be touching, and your lips should barely be touching.

Breathe normally, through your nose, and stay in this relaxed position for about ten minutes. At the end, roll on to your side, slowly open your eyes and allow yourself half a minute or so to come back to the real world before standing up.

Changing relationships

The menopause can often be a time of upheaval in relationships. You are having to learn to treat your children as adults, while with your elderly parents you may have to take on the role of a mother again. At the same time you may also be adjusting to being a grandparent. There may also be the sadness of losing friends of your own generation as well as your own parents.

This is a time when many women begin to look much more critically at their closest relationship – usually the one with their partner. With the children away from home and retirement either on the horizon or already a reality, you may well start to question whether the life you share together is as you want it. We are living longer, and for some couples this could mean a further 30 years together. Increasing numbers of women choose this time of their lives to make a fresh start – either leaving a marriage or relationship or going for a complete overhaul to revitalize what they have. Men, of course, have been leaving their wives at this time in their lives for years, but today's women are less downtrodden and far more outspoken about what they want for themselves.

Not all women leave for another relationship – many leave because they have had enough of sharing their life with another person and long for the freedom that the single life offers. But before you take that decision, you might want to consider marriage guidance or some form of relationship counselling.

I left Alec ten months after my fiftieth birthday. In many ways I know it was a selfish thing to do, but running through my mind had been the constant thought that life is so short, and do I really want to spend my remaining years with this person who I no longer love or respect? It hasn't been as wonderful as I expected – I've been horribly lonely at times and sometimes I wonder what will happen in the future when I am not so active – but looking back I think I probably did the right thing.

This is also a time when you may have to rethink contraception. You may be starting a new relationship and will have to use contraception for the first time in decades especially if your previous partner had a vasectomy. Contraception should be used for two years if your menopause takes place when you are under 50 and for a year if you are over 50. Ask your GP or local family planning clinic for advice. There is a higher percentage of abortions for unwanted pregnancies in the 45–55 age group than in any other.

Sex

During the menopause many women experience problems due to the changes that are taking place in their bodies. Soreness and dryness in the vagina can make sex less than enjoyable and even painful. If left untreated, this can completely undermine any sexual desire. This problem can be solved by using lubrication – various products can be bought over the counter at the chemist, from KY Jelly, a simple water-based lubricant which can be used just before intercourse or as part of foreplay, to Replens (polycarbophil), which you use with an applicator three times a week to reduce atrophy as well as increase lubrication and acidity levels in the vagina. HRT is known to help by increasing the flow of blood to the vagina, and stimulating lubrication and oestrogen creams can also be applied locally.

It is also very common for your emotions to play a part in how you feel about sex. If you feel depressed, tired and lacking in confidence or enthusiasm, it can easily affect your sex life. You will simply not feel in the mood, and if you do make the effort you may find it hard or impossible to be sufficiently aroused to enjoy it. Many women on HRT report that it improves their sex lives – not just because of the reduction in the physical symptoms, but also because of the fact that they begin to feel more positive about themselves.

If your sex life has always been satisfying and you have a good relationship with your partner, you should be able to find ways together to regain the closeness you have shared in the past. Talking about your feelings with your partner – and some understanding on his part that there are times when you simply want to cuddle and caress rather than make love – can help a great deal. If sex has been unsatisfactory in the past or if your relationship is shaky, then the physical and emotional symptoms of the menopause will play a much more important role. If you can talk to each other it will help, or you may find that guidance from a counsellor can help you air the issues that are bothering you.

At the same time, your partner may also be experiencing changes that will affect your sex lives. If he is still at work, he may be under pressure there and this stress can affect his performance in bed. If you know or sense that this may be the problem, then it will help to discuss this between you and perhaps find ways to relax. Although the debate about a male menopause continues, the fact is that it often takes an older man longer to establish an erection and he may not be able to maintain it for as long. It may then take some time before he is ready to make love again. These changes are due to falling levels of testosterone, and while some men can adjust easily, others find it very undermining. Many men do worry about their sexual performance, and one or two unsatisfactory experiences can make them fear that they might be impotent. This can become a self-fulfilling prophecy.

If your partner cannot get an erection or has problems, then try to talk openly together about this. It often makes sense to persuade him to seek medical advice in the early stages, because there can often be a simple explanation. Around a half of all cases of erectile dysfunction are purely psychological, and in this case sex counselling is usually a good option for treatment. Physical reasons for impotence can be due to the side-effects of some drugs, especially some types of beta blocker taken for heart conditions. If this is the case, the doctor can prescribe a different formula. If your partner has diabetes then the nerves that stimulate erections may have been damaged. Poor circulation, especially in the arteries of the legs, will also affect the blood flow to the penis. There are treatments for impotence – Viagra is the best-known medical treatment and it seems to work for women as well. There are also other options such as injections of a drug, papaverine, into the penis, which can help men who have any diseases that affect the blood supply or the nerves. There are also appliances such as vacuum devices which draw blood gently into the penis.

For many women (and their partners) after the menopause, sex is better than ever. In some ways you can rediscover the freedom of youth, with the added bonus of no longer having to worry about contraception or pregnancy. If you are single, your sex life can be equally successful and active, but you will still need to take precautions against infections and AIDS. If you are married there may be more privacy if the children have left home, more time once you are retired. You are no longer constrained to make love in bed, at night, at the end of a long day when you are both tired. A happy, healthy sex life is very like exercise – the more you practise it, the better it becomes.

It is also worth remembering that there are other ways to give each other pleasure apart from full sexual intercourse, and with more time for each other you can enjoy exploring and experimenting together.

6

HRT: is it for you?

Hormone replacement therapy (HRT) is the recognized treatment for a whole range of menopausal symptoms from hot flushes to vaginal dryness. The role of HRT is to replace the missing hormones, chiefly oestrogen, that cause these symptoms. Properly prescribed, so that the dose is right for the individual woman, it can completely revitalize someone suffering from the exhausting symptoms of the menopause.

More interestingly, HRT is also increasingly prescribed for women post-menopause because of the long-term protection it can offer against some of the serious and disabling diseases of later life.

The benefits of HRT

Short-term benefits

There are several reasons why you may want to take HRT. In the first instance, it has been shown to offer effective relief from some of the most uncomfortable symptoms of the menopause – hot flushes, night sweats, painful intercourse caused by a dry vagina, urinary problems, headaches.

In studies, around 90 per cent of women reported that on taking HRT their symptoms had gone altogether, and an even higher proportion of women say that HRT has at least brought them some relief and that their symptoms are less strong.

Higher levels of oestrogen can also benefit your looks by increasing the amount of collagen in the skin, which is why women on HRT may find that their skin remains firmer, with fewer wrinkles. Provided they eat a balanced diet they can also retain their pre-menopausal body shape, keeping a defined waistline and avoiding a bulging stomach. Then there is a general feeling of well-being, emotional stability, a sense of being in control and often a return of lost confidence.

Women also say that they find it easier to concentrate and perform intellectual tasks and that their sleep patterns improve, so that they feel more rested when they wake and their sleep is less disturbed. Women on HRT may also have more satisfying sex lives – this may be linked to solving the problem of vaginal dryness, and it is also believed that HRT may have a direct effect on libido and satiation in the brain. However, it may also be due to the fact that women on HRT do seem to have a more positive approach to life and to the menopause.

These are the main reasons why women at the menopause feel that HRT is well worth taking, but increasingly the treatment's long-term benefits are also being taken into consideration.

Long-term benefits

Declining oestrogen levels at and post-menopause increase a woman's risk of osteoporosis and the disability and pain it can cause. Coronary heart disease is the leading cause of death among women over 50, putting them at the same level of risk as men. It is known that by restoring the declining supply of oestrogen, HRT offers good protection against both these diseases.

The most significant amount of bone loss tends to occur in the first years after the menopause, so to gain the best protection and prevent this bone loss, HRT should ideally be started during the menopause rather than after. However, it is never too late, as a study of older women who started HRT in their later years found that it reduced their risk of hip fractures. Restoring oestrogen can also improve the health of your teeth, gums, hair and nails, making them stronger and less brittle and reducing the chances of periodontal (gum) disease, which can loosen teeth.

Similarly, where heart disease is concerned, HRT appears to act on cholesterol – lowering the levels of LDL, the 'bad' cholesterol, while raising levels of HDL, the 'good' cholesterol.

As research continues, more long-term benefits are being discovered, although more studies need to be carried out. HRT may well delay the onset of Alzheimer's Disease and other problems affecting brain function, may provide some protection against cancers of the colon and the bowel, and may also help prevent the development of Parkinson's Disease. However, there are risks and side-effects associated with taking this treatment and these need to be borne in mind, when you are making your decision.

What is HRT?

Put simply, hormone replacement therapy is the medical treatment for the symptoms of the menopause that occur because of changing hormone levels. HRT replaces the two hormones, oestrogen and progesterone, that the body is making less of at this time.

Declining oestrogen levels produce a whole range of uncomfortable symptoms – hot flushes, vaginal dryness, sleep and urinary problems – which oestrogen replacement can effectively relieve. When HRT was first developed in the USA in the 1950s and brought to Britain in the 1960s, this is what it was principally prescribed for. For many women it seemed to be a miracle as it transformed their lives by getting rid of symptoms that had been a misery.

Subsequent trials have shown that women on HRT suffered from less osteoporosis (brittle bones) and heart disease, and it became clear that the therapy could have much wider benefits.

The hormones used

Oestrogen

Oestrogen is the primary hormone in HRT. Two types can be used, 'natural' oestrogens from human or animal sources (oestradiol, oestrone, equilin, 17alpha-dihydroequilin) and synthetic oestrogens (dienestrol, ethinyloestradiol, mestranol) which are available in a variety of different strengths. The natural oestrogens are similar to the oestrogens the body produces, while the synthetic oestrogens have a similar effect but their structure is different – it is these synthetic oestrogens that are used, in high doses, for the oral contraceptive pill.

When it comes to oestrogen replacement, the dose is lower, and usually natural oestrogen is used to minimize the risks of blood clots forming. Although neither of the oestrogens in HRT is exactly the same as those produced within the body, careful adjustment of the dose can ensure that the body can accept and utilize them properly.

Progesterone

Progesterone, which is always included in HRT given to women who still have a womb, is the other major female hormone. In the 1960s, it was realized that oestrogen taken on its own could thicken the endometrium (womb lining) and increase the risk of developing endometrial cancer. Natural progesterone tablets are difficult to take, because to be really effective they need to be taken several times a day or as a suppository, so a synthetic form was developed called progestogen. The drawback with progestogen is that it normally results in a monthly bleed, although new types (taken continuously in post-menopausal women) can avoid this. Progestogens may also trigger pre-menstrual symptoms in the first few months, although this should settle down. However, for women who have had a hysterectomy, oestrogen can usually be used safely on its own.

Testosterone

Testosterone is the other hormone which is occasionally used in hormone replacement therapy, although it is taken separately. It is also produced by the ovaries and is believed to play an important role in maintaining libido, especially after the menopause. Women who have had surgery that involves the removal of the ovaries as well as the womb often complain of a severely reduced sex drive which even oestrogen replacement cannot seem to help. Often this is because their testosterone levels have fallen dramatically, so for them testosterone HRT may be helpful. Although the levels do fall at menopause, for most women the drop is less extreme and most consultants would feel that any loss of libido is effectively treated with oestrogen HRT.

There have been enough large-scale trials over the past decades to confirm that HRT really is effective, not just for the immediate symptoms of the menopause but also for its long-term benefits. It is the first-choice treatment for prevention of osteoporosis and may increasingly be recommended to protect women from developing coronary heart disease.

When to take HRT

Most women who wish to take HRT will start two or three years before their periods finally cease. This is the time when the symptoms of the menopause are likely to be most troublesome and can really make your life a misery. If you have had an early menopause or a hysterectomy which includes removal of the ovaries (oöphorectomy), then your doctor or consultant will advise you to start HRT as soon as convenient, provided it is safe for you to do so. This way you are less likely to experience the full blast of menopausal systems and are also offered additional protection for your bones and heart.

In fact, you can start HRT at any time – even after the menopause. In this case you will not be taking it to relieve specific symptoms such as hot flushes, but to offer long-term protection against conditions such as osteoporosis or heart disease. Research shows that starting HRT even years after the menopause can still reduce hip fractures.

Once you have started HRT, it is advisable to take it for four to five years in order to gain the full benefits. However, it is becoming clear that protection against some conditions, such as heart disease, is only effective if you continue to take HRT. That is why some women continue on HRT for 10 or 20 years or even longer and more research is needed to ascertain what the long-term effects might be. It is already known that your risk of breast cancer increases after ten years on HRT.

How to take it

HRT can be taken orally as tablets, as a patch or gel (when the hormones are absorbed through the skin), as an implant (a pellet inserted through the skin into the fat of the thigh or abdomen every six months), or delivered locally to the vagina as a ring, cream or pessary. There is also a wide range of different types of HRT available, which means that you do have a choice. If one type of HRT does not suit you, then you can try something a little different. It is because women do not realize (and their doctors may not tell them) that they can try other formulations of HRT that many take the treatment for less than six months and give up after that time or even earlier because of side-effects. Other women who might benefit from the treatment do not take it because they are unsure of how HRT will affect them, think that a monthly bleed is unavoidable or have heard or read scare stories about the possible side-effects.

Usually HRT preparations containing natural oestrogens will be prescribed, as these resemble those the body produces and also tend to have fewer side-effects.

You also have a choice of different combinations in the way oestrogen and progestogen are delivered.

Cyclical method

You take oestrogen on its own every day for 21 days and a combination of oestrogen and progestogen for 12–14 days. You then have seven days without tablets in some preparations or seven placebo (dummy) tablets in others, when your hot flushes may come back. During this time you also experience a monthly bleed, unless you have had a hysterectomy. Discuss this with your doctor, as it is safe to miss out the dummy tablets.

Three-monthly

This method is flexible in the sense that you take the progestogen for 14 days only once every three months – this reduces the withdrawal bleed to four times a year. In some cases the bleeding will get slighter and slighter and eventually you may not experience a bleed at all. This formulation is only successful for women who are already having extremely irregular periods or for whom irregular bleeding will be a problem.

Combined continuous method

You take both oestrogen and a very low dose of progestogen together every day without a break. You may have a withdrawal bleed for a few months but this should stop. If you are taking HRT long-term this is a useful method, but it is only prescribed if you have had a complete year without a period.

There are also various ways in which HRT can be administered.

Tablets

This is still the most common way of taking HRT. If you have had a hysterectomy, you will simply take oestrogen tablets continuously; otherwise you will be prescribed oestrogen but you will have to take progestogen tablets as well.

If you have been used to taking tablets such as contraceptive pills, you will probably adapt quite easily to taking HRT in this way. Some women who don't take pills regularly find it hard to remember to take their tablets – especially in the first few months – and of course this can upset the hormonal balance and you will get breakthrough bleeding. Other women just find it a nuisance. You are more likely to experience side-effects from tablets because they contain a higher dose of hormones to compensate for the fact that they have to pass through the gut and the liver to be metabolized into the body. However, on the positive side, it is easy to stop taking the pills if you are experiencing uncomfortable side-effects and feel that the type of HRT you are taking doesn't suit you.

Patches

Some women prefer this method, as it solves the problem of having to remember to take a pill every day, although some studies have shown that it does not have the same beneficial effect on lowering cholesterol levels as pills. A transdermal patch will deliver an exact amount of the appropriate hormone continuously through the skin and straight into the bloodstream. Because of this the dose is lower, so there is less chance of side-effects. The patch has to be changed every three to four days and is placed on clean, dry skin, which is free of bath oils, body lotion or talcum powder. Ideally it should be on a place where it will not be rubbed or creased. Most women choose the upper buttocks, the abdomen or the inner thigh. If you have a sensitive skin you should change where you place the patch each time. The patch will usually stay on for several days, even if you have a shower or a bath; however, if it does come loose you can put another patch on and know that the same steady dose will be delivered.

Going without the patch for half an hour or so will not have any adverse effects, so you can remove it if you want to go swimming or make love and are worried that the patch might rub off or be seen. When you are sunbathing the patch must be covered, and on a sunbed it must be removed.

If you are taking progestogen you will either have to use two patches for some of the month or opt for the type of HRT which combines the two hormones in a single patch.

Many women prefer patches to tablets because the steady dose of hormone produces fewer side-effects. However, the dose administered through a patch is fixed at specific levels and is therefore more difficult to adjust.

Implants

An oestrogen implant will give you a continuous dose of the hormone for around six months. It involves a small operation, with a local anaesthetic to prevent any pain, and this can be performed in out-patients or in theatre following a hysterectomy or removal of the ovaries. A small cut is made in the skin, the implant is inserted and the wound is closed with either a stitch or tiny pieces of tape (Steristrips), which can be removed quite painlessly after about five days. Implants are very convenient – and take away all the bother of remembering to take a pill or change your patch – but they are difficult to remove, so you need to be sure that the treatment and the dose are right for you. They are often suggested if you need HRT to prevent or treat osteoporosis, because the level of oestrogen delivered is high. Usually implants are oestrogen-only, but if you have a lowered sex drive and this is not responding to oestrogen, additional testosterone may be given as a separate implant.

Creams/pessaries

Creams are very useful if your main symptom of the menopause is vaginal dryness or urinary problems. Oestrogen cream can be rubbed in around the vaginal area or inserted into the vagina with an applicator. The benefits are purely local, so you do not get any of the long-term benefits provided by pills and patches. However, you can use an oestrogen cream, gel or pessary alongside conventional HRT, and if you are not really bothered by hot flushes or night sweats, are at low risk for heart disease and osteoporosis or would simply prefer not to take HRT, this can be a good alternative. Nevertheless, if you are going to use this form of oestrogen over several weeks it may be sensible to take progestogen tablets, as some of the oestrogen will be absorbed into the bloodstream.

Gel

Oestrogen gel is an alternative to HRT and is rubbed in each day into the legs or lower body. It has been popular in France for years but has only recently become available in Britain. It is easy to use and only takes minutes to dry, but you have to be careful not to use any other product on the area for at least an hour.

Intra-uterine device (IUD)

The levornorgestrel IUCD is licensed for contraceptive and heavy period uses, but in some menopause clinics it is being used as the progesterone part of HRT. It is believed that in the future this product will gain a licence for menopause treatment as it allows 'no bleed' HRT for the much younger woman.

Tibolone has been developed to be used only by post-menopausal women. It cannot be used until a year after the last menstrual bleed, and ideally you will be asked to take three cycles of progestogen (for 12 days each) to reduce any risk to the endometrium. Its big advantage is that there is no withdrawal bleeding because it does not stimulate the endometrium. Its other main benefit is to improve the skin quality of the vaginal area, making intercourse more comfortable and lowering the risk of urinary and vaginal infections. It can improve cholesterol levels and reduce the loss of bone. It is also thought to enhance libido, thanks to its androgenic effects. Research is going on into whether it can also offer effective protection against heart disease.

Raloxifene

Raloxifene is one of the new generation of drugs called SERMs (selective (o)estrogen receptor modulators). One of the best known is tamoxifen, the drug that is used to treat breast cancer and to prevent the disease recurring. SERMs have been developed specifically to target certain areas where oestrogen is needed. In the case of raloxifene (available on prescription as Evista) the aim is to prevent osteoporosis in the spine in post-menopausal women. Unlike HRT it has no effect on short-term symptoms such as hot flushes – indeed, it may actually provoke them. It also has the same risk of DVT (deep vein thrombosis) but it does reduce the risk of breast cancer. However, this is only the first of many developments and there is hope that in future drugs of this kind may be able to target other areas.

The side-effects and risks of HRT

Although for many women HRT is the perfect treatment both during and after the menopause, at the moment only around 20 per cent of women currently take it, and most of them only take it for a year or less, although 70 per cent do discuss the option with their doctor or someone else in primary care. It is interesting that the group of women most likely to opt for HRT are female doctors or the wives of doctors – perhaps because they are in a better position not only to know a great deal about HRT but also to have their questions answered.

There are a number of reasons why so many women choose not to take HRT or stop taking it after such a short time. In some cases it will simply be because their menopausal symptoms are very mild and they feel that they can manage quite well without treatment. If you are in this group, although you may quite sensibly choose not to take HRT for your menopausal symptoms, you may still want to investigate starting HRT post-menopause in order to protect your bone strength and reduce your risk of heart disease. If you fall into one of the high-risk groups for these decisions, then you could benefit even more from HRT. If you are not sure whether you are at high risk, your final decision will be helped if you ask for a bone density scan and also a blood pressure check.

Other women may have been brought up to feel that the menopause is something they have to cope with on their own. These women may hesitate even to see their doctor about their symptoms, convinced that seeking help is a sign of weakness.

There is also a large group of women who regard the menopause as a natural stage that all women pass through, and who feel that to take hormones is to deny that and in effect tamper with nature.

Another large number of women do take HRT but stop taking it after weeks or months because of withdrawal bleeding and side-effects such as weight gain and breast tenderness. If you have any of these concerns, it really makes sense to return to the doctor or menopause clinic and make sure that the dose you have been given is right for you. To be really successful, HRT should be tailored to the individual, and there are now enough different formulations and types available to make this possible.

However, the majority of women who might benefit from this treatment are deterred by the possible risks associated with HRT in both the short term and the long term – in particular breast cancer and thromboembolism (a blood clot that forms within a blood vessel but which can sometimes break free and block an artery).

Thousands upon thousands of pieces of research are being carried out into the menopause, HRT and associated areas all the time. Often when results are published they will make the headlines, but the study may be based on a very small sample of people. A few days later, results of another study may totally contradict what has been reported. It is little wonder that women get confused, and even doctors find it hard to keep up to date. In the end, many women seem to decide that it is easier to say no to HRT rather than take any risks or have to put up with further discomfort from side-effects.

You should not take HRT if:

- you have endometrial or breast cancer;
- you have undiagnosed vaginal bleeding;
- you have an undiagnosed breast lump;
- you have an existing thromboembolism;
- you are pregnant.

You may be able to take HRT but should take advice from a specialist and be carefully monitored if you have:

- benign breast disease;
- liver or gall bladder disease;
- fibroids;
- endometriosis or past cancer of the womb;
- varicose veins or a past history of DVT (deep vein thrombosis) or thrombosis;
- otosclerosis (a rare condition in which the small bones in the middle ear harden);
- heart disease.

If you have diabetes or hypertension you should be encouraged to have HRT for its protective benefits for your heart but it will make sense to have your diabetes and blood pressure regularly checked.

Breast cancer

The fear that taking extra oestrogen may lead to breast cancer naturally comes high on most women's lists as a reason for not taking HRT. The first thing to do if you have these concerns is to find out whether you fall into the high-risk category for this type of cancer. If the answer to any of the following questions is 'yes', then you need to discuss any decision to take HRT very carefully with your doctor and weight up the pros and cons. Obviously the more risks you have from the list, the greater your risk of developing breast cancer.

- Are you overweight – i.e. is your body mass index (BMI) high?
- Was your first period early?
- Is there a family history of breast cancer?
- Did you have your first child later than normal?
- Are you experiencing a late menopause?

When you think about the risks associated with breast cancer, bear in mind that at the moment 1 woman in 12 will die of breast cancer but this figure refers to older women – over the age of 75. At the age of 50, the figures are 1 in 56. You need to look at the risks of dying from breast cancer in the context of other risks to your health, such as heart disease.

A large analysis of all the existing studies into the risks of breast cancer associated with HRT came to the conclusion that there was a slightly increased risk over and above that associated with increasing age, and that this risk rose the longer you took HRT. For instance, looking at 1,000 women taking HRT over a period of 20 years, 47 would develop breast cancer after five years on HRT and 57 would develop the disease after 15 years on HRT. However, for those not on HRT the chances of breast cancer were still 45 out of the 1,000.

It is also worth remembering that, in this context, you also have a 1 in 4 risk of developing heart disease and a 1 in 6 risk of a hip fracture, so when making the decision you need to examine your individual circumstances and weight up the benefits and risks in discussion with your doctor.

At the same time, making self-examination of your breasts a regular part of your life will ensure that any changes are picked up early.

Blood clots (deep vein thrombosis)

If you have a deep vein thrombosis (DVT) or have had one recently, you should not take HRT. With DVT a blood clot forms in the deep veins of the leg, and unless it is treated it can dislodge and then travel up to the lungs, creating a pulmonary embolus (PE) or a stroke (if the clot blocks the blood supply to the brain). If the DVT occurred some time ago then you may possibly take HRT, although by simply having one DVT you are at greater than average risk of a second. Your clotting factors, especially Factor V Leiden, should be screened by a haematologist, and the pros and cons of HRT can then be fully discussed. If you have other problems of this kind, such as severe varicose veins, or are overweight or immobile, then you should take HRT with caution making sure that you are tested regularly.

Deep vein thrombosis and long-distance travel

Anyone is at greater risk of clots in the legs on a flight lasting longer than four hours or a coach journey lasting more than eight hours. Here is what to do:

- Take an extra two litres of fluid with you to avoid dehydration.
- Get up and move about every two hours.
- Keep exercising your legs and keep the circulation moving.
- Wear loose comfortable clothing – not tight jeans that cut into the groin.
- Avoid alcohol, as it dehydrates, and sedatives.
- There is no research evidence as yet, but some doctors advise starting a low dose of aspirin two days before you travel. Talk to your doctor first, and if she agrees, take one 75mg aspirin a day with food and continue for two days after the flight. Do not take if you are allergic to aspirin, are on an anti-coagulant drug such as Warfarin, have a known stomach ulcer or are breast-feeding.

Abnormal bleeding

If you have experienced any type of abnormal vaginal bleeding then you will need to have this investigated before starting HRT.

Liver disease

In most forms of HRT, such as tablets, the hormones have to pass through the liver on their way into the bloodstream, and the oestrogens then return to the liver to be destroyed and finally excreted in the urine. If you have or have had any problems with your liver then it would be better to take HRT non-orally, perhaps choosing a patch which delivers HRT straight into the bloodstream.

Fibroids

If you have fibroids at the menopause then you will be relieved to know that declining levels of oestrogen are likely to shrink them. However, HRT may cause them to grow larger and symptoms such as irregular bleeding may return. An ultra-sound scan is a good way of monitoring the size of the fibroids; if they are small you may be able to take HRT, but your progress will need to be carefully watched. If the fibroids do grow large and it is still felt that you are benefiting from HRT, then a hysterectomy may be the solution. After it you will be able to go on to oestrogen-only HRT.

Endometriosis

Endometriosis occurs when the small bits of womb lining that are shed each month during a period end up going backwards up the Fallopian tubes or even spilling into your abdominal cavity. These pieces of tissue grow and form cysts. Every woman has at least some endometriosis, giving pain around period time. Because it is the presence of oestrogen that causes endometriosis, at the menopause these problems will usually subside. HRT can take some women back several stages, and in a small proportion of cases endometriosis will return. You will need to weigh the pros and cons carefully to decide whether the benefits of HRT will outweigh the risk of endometriosis returning.

Gallstones

HRT is known to aggravate gallstones, so if you have had them in the past you may not want to risk having them again. However, if you have had your gall bladder removed then you need not be concerned.

Diabetes

In the past, women with diabetes were advised not to take HRT, but now, with proper monitoring, you may be advised to take it because it can help to lower the increased risk of heart disease caused by diabetes and improve glycaemic control.

The most common side-effects of HRT

It comes as a bit of a shock, when you first start HRT, to discover that although it may alleviate your hot flushes, night sweats and so on, it may also trigger a whole range of new symptoms. The most common are:

- tender breasts;
- nausea;

- stomach cramps;
- bloating;
- breakthrough bleeding;
- insomnia;
- headaches;
- weight gain;
- depression and irritability.

It is often these side-effects that discourage women from persevering with HRT and may even put some women off even trying the treatment. In most cases the side-effects disappear within weeks of starting the treatment, although they may last longer in some cases.

If you are suffering really badly, it could be that you are on the wrong formulation or the wrong dose. There are over 50 different types of HRT on the market today and they deliver different strengths of oestrogen. The cause of most of the side-effects is high levels of oestrogen, so if things don't settle down it may make sense to reduce the dose. It helps to remember that if you are in the early stages of your menopause and still having periods, then your body is still producing some oestrogen, and this could explain high levels, and the side-effects that accompany them. If you are worried that you are gaining weight, you may find that changing to a patch can help you to lose more fluid.

Progestogen causes similar side-effects, and here again you should ask for the dose to be adjusted or choose a different make or method of administering the treatment.

Other medical choices

It may be that you cannot or do not want to take HRT but are still looking for some medical help which does not involve hormones. There are various options, and full details of a natural approach are in Chapter 7.

Clonidine

If you have very uncomfortable hot flushes and cannot take HRT then Clonidine may be helpful. It doesn't work for everybody. It is quite safe to take with active breast cancer.

Paroxetine

This drug is an anti-depressant but very effective against hot flushes. It is quite safe to take if you have or have had breast cancer and are on Tamoxifen.

Mood-altering drugs

In the past it was quite common for doctors to prescribe tranquilliz-ers, sedatives or anti-depressants for women going through the menopause. Of course, it is quite possible to be clinically depressed or suffer from panic attacks or excessive anxiety at any time in your life. The mid forties onwards can be a very stressful time, but feeling depressed and unable to cope are sometimes among the symptoms of the menopause.

However, any mental condition needs to be taken seriously and not just dismissed as being what you must expect 'at this time of life'. If you already have physical symptoms of the menopause, your doctor may suggest taking HRT in the first place and seeing whether this helps at all with your emotional symptoms. If it does not, then suitable drugs (which can be taken alongside HRT or, if you are not taking HRT, on their own) should be offered, together with a programme of counselling or psychotherapy.

Although so much has been written and talked about HRT and vast amounts of time and money spent on research it is still not as widely used as those who developed it probably expected or hoped. Whatever you do decide to do, it needs to be based on knowledge of what is involved. This gives you a chance to weigh things up and see where the risks and benefits are and how they balance out. If the practice nurse at your local surgery runs a dedicated menopause clinic, this is the ideal place to go to ask questions. After that, you are in a much better position to make your own informed decision.

7

The natural approach

Many women are unaware that they do have a choice when it comes to treating the symptoms of the menopause.

If you see your doctor for advice about uncomfortable symptoms of the menopause, you are most likely to be offered HRT as the best solution. If you cannot take HRT for health reasons, or do not wish to take it, there are still doctors today who will tell you that you will just have to put up with your symptoms.

Of course, HRT can be an excellent treatment for some women, particularly if you feel comfortable about taking it and it is doing what it is supposed to do for you. However, if you have tried HRT and had side-effects, or have been told that it would be safer not to take hormone replacements, or if you simply don't like the idea, then you do have other options – natural and complementary ways of treating your menopausal symptoms and taking care of your health.

These ways are often based on traditional remedies. As with HRT, some may work better for you than others, and some may have little effect. There is very little conclusive research about how successful complementary treatments are for menopausal symptoms, and many of the trials that have been carried out use only a relatively small sample of women. These therapies cannot be compared to HRT, which is a targeted medical treatment, but women who have used natural therapies successfully report that it helps them to feel far more in control. Given the strong links between mind and body and the way they can react off each other, it no longer seems far-fetched to suggest that feeling you have your health in your own hands may also help to relieve many physical symptoms.

Some natural therapies can be taken alongside HRT – the treatments are by no means mutually exclusive and can even complement each other. In most cases the natural therapies offer a gentler approach, particularly if you are concerned about the long-term effects of HRT or have found the side-effects unpleasant: most natural therapies, provided they are taken with care, do not carry any risks long-term and there are rarely side-effects.

Herbs and plants themselves are potent, so always keep to the recommended dosage – after all, many of today's drugs were originally derived from plants. Don't imagine because it's 'only a herb' that you can double the dose without any possible side-effects.

If your remedies have been specifically prescribed for you by a qualified practitioner, report back if there are any side-effects or your symptoms are worse, just as you would to your doctor. You should also let your GP know if you plan to use alternative or complementary treatments to alleviate symptoms of the menopause.

What to choose

A natural approach to the menopause can cover a whole range of therapies. Choose the ones that are right for you, those you feel comfortable with and that seem to suit your personality and lifestyle. Whether you decide to take just a single herbal remedy or draw on a whole range of different therapies, the choice is yours.

Don't expect instant results. In most cases herbal remedies and other treatments take time to have an effect – often it will take at least a month and sometimes three months before you notice any real difference.

Here are some of the complementary therapies that seem to work well for many women at the menopause – and what they can help with most. Before you place yourself in the hands of any therapist, use the following guidelines:

- Always see a qualified practitioner – some therapies now have umbrella organizations that can give you a list of practitioners in your area.
- Make sure that the person you see belongs to a recognized organization and has appropriate insurance.
- Because complementary therapists treat everyone as an individual, taking into account your past medical and personal history as well as your present symptoms, it is often worth seeing someone for an initial consultation. If you feel comfortable with them you can return; if not, then you have not over-committed yourself.

This is especially true of herbal or homoeopathic remedies. It is possible to buy these over the counter in most chemists and health food shops, but a practitioner will be able to offer a remedy specifically tailored for you.

You are what you eat

This is a time when it is even more important to eat well (see p. 69). A nutritional therapist will look at your current diet and make sure the balance is correct. The focus will often be on whether there are any shortages in vitamins and minerals and whether there may be foods that you are not tolerating as well as you think.

What can help

Elsewhere in the world a diet with less meat but with more vegetables and fruit and an increased intake of fibre seems to help women to pass more smoothly through the menopause. In Japan fewer than 10 per cent of women suffer from hot flushes (whereas the figure over here is nearer 80 per cent); although a positive mental attitude towards the menopause may play a part, it is far more likely that the answer lies in their diet, which traditionally is high in soya foods such as tofu and miso and low in fat.

Phyto-oestrogens

These are plant oestrogens that occur naturally in many foods but particularly in soya, red clover and linseed and also in other beans, seeds and nuts.

Phyto-oestrogens are very similar to human oestrogen but less powerful. Research in Australia, reported in the *British Medical Journal* in 1990, revealed that a group of menopausal women who regularly ate food high in phyto-oestrogens were able to resolve the problem of dry vagina just as well as a group of women on HRT. This first study was followed by others and has allowed us to understand why Japanese women experience so few symptoms of the menopause. One of the main differences in the Japanese diet is the high level of phyto-oestrogens, mainly from soya and soy products. In fact there is no word in Japanese for 'hot flushes'. Japanese women also experience a much lower incidence of breast cancer, heart disease and hip fractures caused by osteoporosis. Yet when they leave their own country to live in the West and eat a normal Western diet, their risks of experiencing all or any of the conditions mentioned above increase.

Phyto-oestrogens are only found in plants, but the oestrogen component is easily absorbed into the body and circulated round in the blood and tissues. There are over a thousand different chemical sub-groups within phyto-oestrogens, all with a similar chemical structure to human oestrogen. Attention has focused on a group called the isoflavones, found mainly in beans (especially soya), linseeds, chick peas, lentils, sprouting seeds such as alfalfa and aduki beans. Four isoflavones in particular – genistein, daidzein, formono-netin and biochanin – have caught everyone's interest: they are believed to offer women protection against hormonally related diseases such as breast cancer, heart disease and osteoporosis.

Although phyto-oestrogens are so similar to oestrogen, they are much weaker and are usually referred to as 'weak SERMS'. They have a balancing effect on our hormone levels. During the menopause, while the body is still producing oestrogen they may prevent it from producing too much, but when levels are low they can give it a boost. This action can also reduce the effect of oestrogen surges, such as hot flushes and dizziness. In one study, women reported a reduction of over 40 per cent in hot flushes. Phyto-oestrogens also seem to improve cholesterol levels by raising the levels of HDL – the 'good' cholesterol – and lowering those of LDL, the 'bad' cholesterol.

Following the menopause, the same isoflavones have a role as an oestrogen provider, making sure that some oestrogen is still around. As a result, research figures show that, in a similar way to HRT, there is a slight improvement in bone density and some protection against breast cancer and heart disease. Phyto-oestrogens may also lower the risk of prostate cancer, so there is no harm in giving this diet to your partner and children too.

Increasing phyto-oestrogens in your diet

Start by increasing the amount of phyto-oestrogens in your diet. Soya is quite versatile. Apart from TVP (textured vegetable protein), a meat substitute, there are tempeh (fermented soya bean paste) and tofu (soya bean curd). Both have virtually no flavour but can be used in casseroles and stir fries or even threaded on to skewers with other vegetables for kebabs. You can also drink soya milk, sprinkle soya flakes on your morning cereal or make miso (soya bean paste) into a soup. In Japan the average daily intake of isoflavones is around 75 to 100mg – a serving of tempeh or soya milk contains around 40mg. A daily slice of Linda Kearn's 'menopause cake' (see below) will give you all the isoflavones you need.

Many everyday foods are good sources of phyto-oestrogens, so you don't need to make a major change to your diet to include them.

- *Vegetables* such as broccoli, red onions, celery, sweet red peppers, tomatoes, garlic.
- *Fruits* all the berries, grapes (especially red), citrus fruit, plums.
- *Cereals* – barley, couscous, rye, oats, polenta.
- *Seeds and pulses* – sunflower, sesame and pumpkin seeds; chickpeas, haricot and kidney beans, broad beans, lentils.

If you want to take an isoflavone supplement, you should take no more than 50 to 110mg a day. Red clover, black kohosh and dong quai (which is particularly helpful for heavy periods) are considered to be good choices. There are also soy supplements, but although these are high in phyto-oestrogens they are not as high in isoflavones.

Some root vegetables – carrots, beetroot, parsnips, sweet potatoes – and pulses such as chickpeas, as well as providing plant oestrogens, can help the body to produce its own progesterone.

To help reduce hot flushes some women find it helps to increase their intake of vitamin E, either from foods such as blackberries, avocado, nuts and seeds – sunflower or pumpkin – or through supplements such as evening primrose oil or starflower oil.

If you see a nutritional therapist, you will probably be advised to take a variety of vitamin and/or mineral supplements, on the basis of your symptoms and your overall health. If you are treating yourself then the following supplements can be helpful:

- magnesium and vitamin B complex for irritability and anxiety;
- magnesium for sleep problems and to improve your libido;
- co-enzyme Q10 for extra energy;
- vitamin C with bioflavanoids for hot flushes/night sweats;
- zinc for healthy skin;
- vitamin E for vaginal dryness. Some practitioners recommend inserting a vitamin E capsule into the vagina, as this is more effective than taking it orally.

Linda Kearn's 'Beat the Menopause Cake'
Linda Kearn was only 39 when her ovaries were removed. She then took HRT for 13 years. The treatment was never quite right for her, and when she had a breast cancer scare she decided enough was enough. Always a wholefood eater, she knew about the advantages of phyto-oestrogens and developed a special flapjack-type cake based on nuts, seeds and raisins, as well as oats and spices, to cope with some of her symptoms, especially hot flushes. Her 'Beat the Menopause Cake', a sort of flapjack made with seeds as well as grains, worked for other women too and is now available by mail order (see Wellfoods in Useful Addresses, p. 116).

The Eastern approach

The principles of Chinese and other Eastern therapies tend to be preventive. Many women find that traditional Chinese medicine

(TCM) can help symptoms. In TCM, symptoms such as hot flushes, night sweats and tiredness are believed to be caused initially by the decline in reproductive energy. Although erratic periods can affect the blood and liver, the main organs involved are the kidneys, and most remedies will focus on restoring energy to that area.

Natural progesterone

This skin cream is often marketed as an alternative to HRT. The cream is rubbed into the skin so that it is absorbed straight into the bloodstream. It is made by a chemical process synthesizing the product from either wild yam or soya beans. Trials into its efficacy are continuing, and many women report a reduction in hot flushes and night sweats. There are claims that it can also improve bone density, but trials for the National Osteoporosis Society at the Chelsea and Westminster Hospital in London have still to be completed. In the meantime, it is worth remembering that although the body continues to produce some oestrogen throughout a woman's life, the production of progesterone stops completely at the menopause, so it might be safer, if you want to use the cream, not to use it long-term until its safety has been confirmed. It is not thought to provide endometrial protection if you are using conventional oestrogen HRT. It is best to consult your doctor about this.

Herbal remedies

Herbs have been used to cure and treat a whole range of conditions for thousands of years. Many of today's drugs, such as aspirin from willow bark and digitalis from foxglove, have been developed from herbs and plants. The remedies you buy over the counter in the chemist or health food store use the whole plant rather than an extract of the most powerful elements, so they tend to be free from side-effects.

Whatever herbal remedy you choose, be careful to keep to the prescribed dose. If you are buying your herbal remedies over the counter you may well find combinations of some of the herbs mentioned below which you can take to alleviate a number of different symptoms. Always read the labels carefully, and if you are already on prescribed medication mention this to the herbalist or pharmacist to make sure there are no adverse reactions.

If you have a very particular problem you will probably benefit from seeing a qualified herbalist, who will be able to prescribe something specific, taking into consideration your overall health. This will quite often be a combination of different herbs. If you are prescribed several different herbs, you may be advised to take them at different times of the day.

Best herbs for the menopause

- *Dong quai (Chinese angelica)* is often used for a whole range of menstrual problems but can also be quite effective for peri-menopause symptoms such as irregular periods and period pains. Some women also find it relieves hot flushes, night sweats and vaginal dryness.
- *Black kohosh, false unicorn root, agnus castus and liquorice* are all believed to help balance the hormones and so may reduce symptoms such as hot flushes and night sweats.
- *Hops and valerian* can help relieve insomnia.
- *Hypericum (St John's Wort)* is well known as an anti-depressant. In Germany doctors now prescribe it more frequently than anti-depressant drugs, and it certainly seems to help many women overcome mild to moderate depression. It also reduces feelings of fatigue where there is no obvious physical cause. In a small study on 11 women with menopausal symptoms, 60 per cent reported that they had regained their libido, over 60 per cent suffered fewer headaches and less lack of concentration, and by the end of the study 80 per cent felt that their symptoms had improved considerably or gone altogether. However, if you are on any other prescribed medication you should check with your doctor before taking hypericum, as it does produce occasional reactions with standard drugs.
- *Sage and vervain* can both help you to deal with tension and stress.
- *Evening primrose oil* may be useful for pre-menstrual stress and also to help relieve a dry vagina.
- *Calendula cream and pure aloe vera juice* may also be suggested for external use to help vaginal dryness or irritation.
- *Ginseng* is often prescribed to give you more energy and also enable you to deal better with stress. It is believed to regulate hormones.
- *Yarrow* can lower body temperature, so it may help to reduce hot flushes and night sweats.
- *Motherwort* is a good remedy for soothing jangled nerves, helping

you to sleep better and reducing vaginal dryness. It is most effective if you take it as a tincture several times a day – a dozen drops in a little water.

Homoeopathy

Homoeopathy treats like with like. Minute doses are given to produce the same symptoms as those you are experiencing, with the aim of cancelling them out: the body's healing systems are encouraged to fight their own battle. There are a number of homoeopathic remedies that are recommended for specific symptoms of the menopause. Sepia is frequently used to treat hot flushes, headaches and irritability. Although you can buy many remedies over the counter, the range is huge – there are 2,000 different remedies available – so if there seems to be no change in your symptoms you might want to have a consultation with a homoeopath. During the first visit she will talk to you about your immediate symptoms but she will also be interested in your past medical history, both physical and emotional, your lifestyle, your moods. She will then be in a position to prescribe a remedy that is appropriate for you.

It is sometimes possible to see a homoeopath on the NHS.

Acupuncture

Acupuncture is an essential part of traditional Chinese medicine and is used alongside more modern medicine in countries like China. It is based on the idea that the body's energy, or 'chi', needs to be in perfect balance in order for you to be in good health. The chi has two qualities – yin and yang. Yin is female (its qualities are cold and rest) and yang is male (with the qualities of heat and energy). Chi flows through the twelve channels (called meridians) that link up with specific areas of the body; by inserting very fine needles in specific places, the flow can be adjusted and the balance of energy between yin and yang restored. A lot of women find regular acupuncture sessions really helpful during the menopause simply because fluctuating hormones are causing an imbalance.

Acupuncture is regularly used to treat a whole range of menopausal symptoms and conditions. You may find that it simply helps you to feel better in yourself – reducing stress and insomnia – or you may want to use it specifically for pain relief or for chronic conditions such as migraine or arthritis. It is important to be treated by a fully qualified practitioner (see Useful Addresses, p. 115).

Shiatsu

Shiatsu, sometimes called acupressure, is a Japanese therapy in which the practitioner uses her hands, fingers and sometimes her elbows or knees to stimulate the points along the energy channels. Different levels of pressure are used depending on what needs to be treated. Shiatsu is particularly good for relieving insomnia, headaches and anxiety. Although it's best to see a qualified practitioner, you can practise the therapy yourself or get a partner or friend to treat you. Many women like Shiatsu because there is no need to undress or even lie down – the therapy can be performed while sitting in a straight-backed chair.

Massage and essential oils

There are all types of massage available these days – Swedish, Thai, Indian head massage, to name just three.

Massage has been shown to be beneficial for all sorts of conditions and is now routinely used in several hospitals as a way to help patients cope better with pain or uncomfortable treatments and tests.

Psychologically, having someone place their hands on you in a healing way can be very useful at this time. It can help you to feel calmer, more accepting, better about yourself. By helping you to relax and release tension, massage encourages better sleep patterns and may help reduce your feelings of irritability.

Headaches and pains in muscles and joints respond well to massage. Very often head, neck and shoulder pains are due to tension; as the area is massaged, the muscles can relax. In a similar way, stiff, painful joints or soft tissue injuries can be gently massaged to restore movement.

Aromatherapy massages can be used to treat all sorts of complaints from hot flushes to painful periods. A qualified therapist will be able to mix a blend of essential oils to suit your condition, and part of the treatment will involve inhaling these oils as they are massaged into your body. The oils recommended particularly for the menopause include sandalwood, rose and fennel, but many other oils can be effective for symptoms such as depression and mood swings.

Using the oils at home

Essential oils can also be used at home. If you are planning a massage it is very important to dilute your chosen oil or oils with a base oil such as almond, grapeseed or sesame. Essential oils can be added to a bath but only after all the water has been run in. If you want them to disperse better you can mix them with a tablespoon of base oil or even a cup of fresh milk. To get the most from the bath, have a wash or shower first so you can use the bath simply for relaxation.

For headaches try an inhalation, adding four or five drops of essential oil to a pint of near boiling water in a small bowl. Use a towel large enough to cover your head and the bowl, close your eyes and breathe in the scented steam for about five minutes. To reduce the risk of scalding yourself should the bowl be knocked over, place your small bowl inside a larger bowl.

Use a vaporizer to soothe and relax, especially in the evening: a few drops of lavender in some water in a shallow dish over a nightlight will last for about two hours and prepare you for a good night's sleep.

Choose a massage that you feel comfortable with and make sure the therapist is qualified. Some women love a full body massage, others prefer to focus on neck and shoulders. Most therapists will adapt their massage to suit your needs, and that also means that you can ask for a massage to be firmer or more gentle. Sometimes working on a particularly tense area such as the shoulders can be quite uncomfortable, so it's up to you to say if it's too much.

Self-massage

Often you can get relief and relaxation and boost energy levels with self-massage – it also helps you feel more in control. It's instinctive anyway to rub a place that hurts, and massage simply extends this.

A face and head massage can do wonders to soothe a stressful headache. You can either sit in a chair or lie down on the floor. Close your eyes and do the movements purely by touch.

- Placing your hands on either side of your face, gently stroke all over.
- Use your fingers to make small and then large circles all over your face and forehead, applying extra pressure as you return to each area, especially around the jaw where there is often tension.
- Cup your palms over your ears and listen to the soothing sound of the sea.

- Place your hands flat on your forehead, fingers touching, and draw them gently apart until the fingers reach the temples. Stop there and press gently. Repeat several times.
- Run your fingers slowly and smoothly through your hair, making sure you start at the roots. Let one hand follow the other without a pause.

Reflexology

This form of massage focuses just on the feet and has many elements from acupuncture and acupressure. Reflexologists work on the principle that all the major organs of the body have corresponding areas in the feet. By feeling these various areas a therapist can tell whether certain areas or organs are out of balance and need treatment.

The treatment itself will involve a mixture of massage and pressure applied on specific points of the foot. The therapy suits a lot of people who prefer not to have to take their clothes off, and the treatment itself is very relaxing, although there can be moments of discomfort when the therapist puts pressure on certain points.

Like other forms of massage, reflexology is good for easing emotional tension, and many people report relief from conditions such as migraines and high blood pressure, skin conditions such as psoriasis and digestive problems such as irritable bowel syndrome.

T'ai chi and yoga

Although T'ai chi comes from China and yoga comes from India, both offer similar spiritual and physical benefits.

T'ai chi has its roots in the martial arts, with the aim of using minimum force to fight aggression. The Yang style most generally practised today was developed in the early twentieth century. Jumps, kicks and punches have been eliminated so the focus is on health, stimulating the flow of chi (energy) round the body. Once you have learned some of the movements of T'ai chi (the 'forms') you will find that together they create a set, with each form flowing gracefully into the next. The whole session then becomes almost a meditation, in which you focus on making each move and performing it as well as you can. The movements themselves are not complicated, but they are very controlled and slow so they are excellent for strengthening muscles in the legs, arms, abdomen and back and for maintaining balance and co-ordination. Correct breathing is also involved, to help relaxation and make the best use of energy.

Yoga follows a similar path, with a variety of different asanas (postures). Like T'ai chi it is non-competitive; you simply perform each asana to the best of your ability. Yoga is a wonderful way to strengthen, stretch and improve flexibility and balance, but it also works on the mind, helping to relieve stress and anxiety. With relaxation can come a drop in high blood pressure, better sleep and improved digestion. You need a certain amount of stamina for yoga but you can build this up over time. Most classes should start with a few minutes of meditation to clear the mind, followed by some pranayama (breathing exercises) which help you to focus on the asanas as well as relaxing the body.

Because the asanas are static there is a very low risk of injury, but you should always tell your yoga teacher if you have a structural problem such as a knee injury or back pain.

Classes for yoga are very easy to find, and T'ai chi classes are now more widely available. Once the movements and postures have been learned and you know how to perform them correctly, they can both be practised at home on your own at a time that suits you.

I had wanted to try yoga for many years, and as I reached my late forties it seemed the right time. I found a local class with a really wonderful teacher. She was very careful to check each time in case someone had a back problem or a sore knee – in fact, anything that might be injured. Then she would come round and adjust our position so that it was absolutely right. It was so different from the aerobic classes I'd gone to a decade before. Some of the asanas seemed quite easy, but you were always encouraged to stretch just that bit further, to hold the pose a little longer. What I particularly like is the fact that you have this inner focus – there's no time to look at what anyone else is doing and compare techniques, you are totally absorbed in what you are doing. As a result it's wonderfully relaxing – a whole hour when you can't think of anything else but what you are doing at that precise moment. And of course I love the deep relaxation at the end of each session.

Back and joint problems

While back and joint problems may not be a particular feature of the menopause, they inevitably increase as we get older. Three therapies are especially helpful.

Chiropractic

Chiropractic works on the belief that the spine influences problems in other parts of the body, so if the spine is properly aligned it can relieve other conditions such as digestive problems, as well as conditions more directly related to the spine such as headaches and muscle and joint pain. Before starting any treatment a chiropractor will take a full medical history and ask you questions about your lifestyle. To help with the diagnosis, X-rays may be taken. The first treatment session will last up to an hour, but as the condition improves the sessions will be shorter.

Osteopathy

Osteopathy differs from chiropractic in that not just the spine but also the muscles, joints and bones are involved in the treatment. An osteopath will take a thorough medical history and include questions about how you feel emotionally. She may use massage, stretching or manipulation techniques to treat a range of problems. The therapy is particularly successful for back pain, including sciatica and sports injuries.

Alexander Technique

This is a useful therapy if you are experiencing back or joint pain. It teaches improved posture; even standing and sitting correctly can do wonders, not just for chronic back pain but for other conditions too, as all the organs have more space to function efficiently. Learning to move gracefully and naturally again, as you did as a child, and casting aside bad habits such as slumping can also improve self-esteem and self-confidence. As you walk you hold yourself tall and look the world in the eye. Most classes are individual, and you practise what you are taught at home.

Using natural remedies for menopausal symptoms involves thinking quite carefully about how you feel and what your needs are. It demands a greater degree of involvement with your body and mind and what's happening to them than you might have when you take a prescribed medicine. The holistic approach means that the whole person is being treated. Many women report improvements in physical symptoms, but you may also gain psychological benefits. Feeling more in control can help you to view this stage in your life as an entirely natural process rather than an illness that has to be treated or a deficiency that has to be corrected.

A natural approach to the menopause doesn't mean you have to turn your back on orthodox medicine. There may well be times when medical treatment is necessary. It is important to continue to see your GP to check out any unusual symptoms such as abnormal bleeding, possible vaginal infections, breast pain or lumps or frequent headaches, for regular checks on blood pressure and for any screening.

For many of the familiar symptoms of the menopause, orthodox medicine and complementary treatments are increasingly beginning to work comfortably together, and each has something to offer you as you pass through this phase of your life.

Useful Addresses

Note on using the Internet

The Internet has a wealth of information about the menopause and everything associated with it. Just type in 'menopause' and your chosen search engine will probably come up with tens of thousands of possibilities. To narrow the search, be more specific in what you want to know. Always be a little wary of information on a website, as not all sites are completely up-to-date and details may not have been checked or contributed by qualified doctors. Advice or treatments on US, European or Australasian sites may not be available in the UK. For information that you can trust, choose well-established sites that will often be linked to medical organizations, universities or colleges.

Action on Smoking and Health (ASH) UK
102 Clifton Street
London EC2A 4HW
Tel.: 020 7739 5902
www.ash.org

Alcohol Concern
Drinkline: 0800 917 82 82 (freephone)
www.alcoholconcern.co.uk
For support and advice on all problems to do with alcohol

The Amarant Trust
Sycamore House
5 Sycamore Street
London EC1Y 0SG
Menopause and HRT helpline: 0891 660620
Advice line: 01293 413000
Amarant Clinic: 020 7401 3855
For information on HRT

Breast Cancer Care
Kiln House
210 New King's Road
London SW6 4NZ
Tel.: 020 7384 2984 for information on regional offices
Helpline: 0808 800 6000
www.breastcancercare.org.uk
For advice and support on breast cancer and breast care

Breast Care Campaign
Blythe Hall
100 Blythe Road
London W14 0HB
www.breastcare.co.uk

British Association for Counselling
1 Regent Place
Rugby
Warwickshire CV21 2PJ
Tel.: 01788 578328
Information line: 01788 550899

British Heart Foundation
14 Fitzhardinge Street
London W1H 4DH
Tel.: 020 7935 0185
www.bhf.org.uk
Send an sae for leaflets on heart health

The Continence Foundation
307 Hatton Square
16 Baldwin's Gardens
London EC1N 7RJ
Helpline: 020 7831 9831
www.continence-foundation.org.uk
For confidential advice and support on incontinence

The Daisy Network
PO Box 2829
Blandford Forum DT11 8YT
The Daisy Chain is a support group for women suffering premature
menopause (before the age of 40) due to ovarian failure or removal

Digestive Disorders Foundation
3 St Andrew's Place
London NW1 4LB
020 7486 0341
www.digestivedisorders.org.uk
For leaflets on conditions such as irritable bowel syndrome, constipation,
wind, etc.

Health Information Service
Tel.: 0800 66 55 44
A national service that has local centres and offers information on a wide
range of health-related issues

Hysterectomy Association
PO Box 27
West Drayton
Middlesex UB7 0SE
or
Aynsley House
Chester Gardens
Church Gresley
Swadlincote
Derbyshire DE11 9PU
www.hysterectomy-association.org.uk/index.htm

The National Endometriosis Society
Suite 50, Westminster Palace Gardens
1–7 Artillery Row
London SW1P 1RL
Tel.: 020 7222 2781
HelpLine: 020 7222 2776

National Osteoporosis Society
PO Box 10
Radstock
Bath BA3 3YB
Tel.: 01761 471771
Helpline: 01761 472721
www.nos.org.uk

Natural Menopause Helpline
228 Muswell Hill Broadway
London N10 3SH
Helpline: 0845 603 1021 (all calls charged at local rate)
Send A4 sae for information

NHS Smoking Helpline
Helpline: 0800 169 0 169

Quit
Helpline: 0800 00 22 00
For giving up smoking

The Pennell Initiative
Tel.: 0161 275 2908
For leaflets on positive steps for later life

Relate
Herbert Gray College
Little Church Street
Rugby
Warwickshire CV21 3AP

Tel.: 01788 563 816 for books on relationships
www.relate.org.uk
See telephone directory for your nearest centre for counselling

TENA Advice Line
Helpline: 0845 30 80 80 30
www.tenalady.co.uk
For information and leaflets on pelvic floor exercises and incontinence
supplies

Thrush Advice Bureau
PO Box 8762
London SW7 4ZD
Tel.: 020 7285 5520
www.thrushadvice.org

Women's Health
52 Featherstone Street
London EC1Y 8RT
Tel.: 020 7251 6333
Helpline: 020 7251 6580
www.womenshealthlondon.org.uk

Women's Health Concern
93–99 Upper Richmond Road
Putney
London SW15 2TQ
Helpline: 020 8780 3007
www.womens-health-concern.org
Telephone the helpline for contact numbers of specialist nurses who will
discuss a whole range of women's health subjects

Women's Nutritional Advisory Service (WNAS)
PO Box 268
Lewes
East Sussex BN7 2QN
Tel.: 01273 487366
Advice and information on natural methods of managing the menopause

WellBeing
(Royal College of Obstetricians and Gynaecologists)
27 Sussex Place
Regent's Park
London NW1 4SP
Tel.: 020 7262 5337
www.wellbeing.org.uk
For leaflets on the menopause and hysterectomy

Eire

Dublin Well Woman Centre
73 Lower Leeson Street
Dublin 2
Tel.: (01) 610 083

Women's Health
35 Lower Liffey Street
Dublin 1
Tel.: (01) 728 051

BreastCheck programme. The register only includes 86 per cent of the women who should be screened so you can register yourself by ringing the helpline on 1800 45 45 55

USA

Hysterectomy Educational Resources and Services
422 Bryn Mawr Avenue
Bala Cynwyd
PA 19004
Tel.: (601) 667 7757
email: HERSfdn@aol.com
HERS is a non-profit organization which provides information about alternatives to hysterectomy

National Osteoporosis Foundation
1232 22nd Street N.W.
Washington, D.C. 20037-1292
Tel.: (202) 223 2226

North American Menopause Society
PO Box 94527
Cleveland
Ohio
OH 44101
Helpline: (900) 370 6267

Canada

The Canadian Continence Foundation
PO Box 30V
Victoria Branch
Westmount
Quebec H3Z 2V4
Tel.: (800) 265 9575/(514) 488 8379

Osteoporosis Society of Canada
National Office
33 Laird Drive
Toronto, Ontario
M4G 3S9
Tel: (416) 696 2663
Email: osc@osteoporosis.ca

Society of Obstetricians and Gynaecologists of Canada
Menopause Helpline: (888) 875 9800

Australia

AMARANT
National Menopause Foundation
Private Bag No. 1
Darlinghurst
NSW 2010
Tel.: (02) 9968 3706

Continence Foundation of Australia
AMA House
293 Royal Parade
Parkville
VIC 3052
Tel.: (03) 9347 2522
Fax.: (03) 9347 2533
Email: contfound.org.au
National Continence Helpline: 1800 33 00 66 (8 a.m.–8 p.m. Monday–
Friday)

The Jean Hailes Medical Centre for Women
291 Clayton Road
Clayton
VIC 3168
Tel.: (03) 9562 7555

Osteoporosis Foundation of Australia
100 Miller Street
27th Floor
North Sydney
NSW 2060
Tel.: (02) 957 5162

New Zealand

New Zealand Continence Association
PO Box 270
Drury, Auckland
Tel.: (09) 294 7738

Email: jannzca@ihug.co.nz
www.continence.org.nz
Bladder Control Helpline: 0800 650 659

Osteoporosis New Zealand
PO Box 688
Wellington
Tel.: (04) 499 4862
Email: info@osteoporosis.org.nz

Women's Health Action
27 Gillies Avenue
Newmarket, Auckland
Tel.: (09) 520 5295
Email: womenh@ihug.co.nz
www.womens-health.org.nz

Complementary therapies

Association of Reflexologists
27 Old Gloucester Street
London WC1N 3XX
Tel.: 0870 567 3320
www.reflexology.org

British Acupuncture Council
63 Jeddo Road
London W12 9HQ
Tel.: 020 8735 0400
www.acupuncture.org.uk

British Wheel of Yoga
1 Hamilton Place
Boston Road
Sleaford
Lincolnshire NG34 7ES
Tel.: 01529 306851
www.members.aol.com/wheelyoga

General Chiropractic Council
344–354 Gray's Inn Road
London WC1X 8BP
Tel.: 020 7713 5155
www.gcc-uk.org
For information on chiropractic and details of qualified practitioners

International Federation of Aromatherapists
182 Chiswick High Road
London W4 1PP
Tel.: 020 8742 2605
www.int-fed-aromatherapy.co.uk

National Institute of Medical Herbalists
56 Longbrook Street
Exeter
Devon EX4 6AH
Tel.: 01392 426022
www.btinternet.com/~nimh/

Osteopathic Information Service
Osteopathy House
176 Tower Bridge Road
London SE1 3LU
Tel.: 020 7357 6655
www.osteopathy.org.uk
For information on osteopathy and advice on qualified practitioners

The Society of Homoeopaths
4a Artizan Road
Northampton NN1 4HU
Tel.: 01604 621400
www.homoeopathy-soh.org.uk

The Society of Teachers of Alexander Technique
20 London House
266 Fulham Road
London SW10 9EL
Tel.: 020 7284 3338
www.stat.org.uk

UK T'ai Chi Association
PO Box 157
Bromley
Kent BR1 3XX
Tel.: 020 8289 5166

Wellfoods Ltd
Unit 6
Mapplewell Business Park
Mapplewell
Barnsley S75 6BP
Tel.: 01226 381 712
www.bake-it.com
For Linda Kearn's cake

Yoga for Health
Ickwell Bury
Biggleswade
Bedfordshire SG18 9EF
Tel.: 01767 627271
www.yogaforhealthfoundation.co.uk

Index